Psychiatry and the CIA: Victims of Mind Control

Psychiatry and the CIA: Victims of Mind Control

Harvey M. Weinstein, M.D.

Director,
Cowell Student Health Center,
Stanford University

American Psychiatric Press, Inc.

Washington, DC
London, England

Books published by the American Psychiatric Press, Inc., represent the views and opinions of the individual authors and do not necessarily represent the policies and opinions of the Press or the American Psychiatric Association.

A previous edition of this book was published in Canada under the title *A Father, a Son and the CIA* (Toronto: James Lorimer & Company, 1988).

All patients' names used in this book are pseudonyms. Some clinical vignettes are composites of several patients.

Manufactured in the United States of America
90 91 92 93 4 3 2 1

American Psychiatric Press, Inc.
1400 K Street, N.W., Washington, DC 20005

The paper used in this publication meets the minimum requirements of the American National Standard for Information Sciences—Permanence of Paper for Printed Library Materials ANSI Z39.48-1984. ♾

Library of Congress Cataloging-in-Publication Data

Weinstein, Harvey.
Psychiatry and the CIA : victims of mind control / Harvey M. Weinstein.
p. cm.
Rev. ed. of: A father, a son and the CIA. 1988.
Includes bibliographical references.
Includes index.
ISBN 0-88048-363-6 (alk. paper)
1. Brainwashing—Québec (Province)—Montréal. 2. Cameron, Ewen, 1901–1967. 3. Allan Memorial Institute. 4. United States. Central Intelligence Agency. 5. Human experimentation in psychology—Québec (Province)—Montréal. 6. Psychiatric ethics—Québec (Province)—Montréal. [1. Cameron, Ewen, 1901–1967. 2. United States. Central Intelligence Agency. 3. Ethics, Medical. 4. Human Experimentation. 5. Persuasive Communication.] I. Weinstein, Harvey. Father, a son and the CIA. II. Title.
[DNLM: BF 637.P4 W424p]
BF633.W45 1990
353.0089—dc20
DNLM/DLC
for Library of Congress 90-707
CIP

British Library Cataloguing in Publication Data

A CIP record is available from the British Library.

For
Bertha Gertsman Weinstein
1907–1981
"A woman of valor"

Contents

Part 3: The Fight

Part 4: The Aftermath

Foreword

Harvey Weinstein's moving description of the destructive experiments carried out on his father by Ewen Cameron has significance that extends far beyond that family tragedy. Cameron was one of the world's most prominent psychiatrists at the time, and his professional corruption was associated with claims of scientific omnipotence, an alliance with cold war intelligence operations, and a quest for personal glory.

What enabled Cameron to go as far as he did was not only his personal authoritarianism but the larger ideologies of "higher purpose" that he and so many others embraced. Killing or maiming human beings on a substantial scale always involves a claim to virtue. Cameron could inwardly justify his participation in immoral CIA-sponsored experiments as contributing to the cure of mental illness, to the struggle against the Communist threat, or to the prevention of the kind of thinking that led to Nazism.

I have found that people tend to be vulnerable to destructive, even genocidal, ideologies when they are able to experience these ideologies as a cure for painful historical trauma they have undergone. In Cameron's case, there was a double trauma: that of Nazi mass murder, and that of the emergence of Communist "brainwashing." From the time he was called upon to examine Rudolf Hess at Nuremberg and thereby immerse himself in Nazi crimes, Cameron tended to connect his interest in behavior control with the combating of Nazi-like tendencies in people. But the more significant trauma for him was his subsequent encounter with Communist efforts at mind control.

I can remember the mixture of horror and fascination evoked by Chinese Communist psychological manipulation of American soldiers captured in Korea. At the end of my own tour of duty with the Air Force, I was one of a team of military psychiatrists assigned to interview these returning prisoners of war, and I was later able to conduct a systematic study of both Westerners and Chinese subjected to a more profound version of the process the Chinese themselves called "thought reform."

That process was of considerable psychological interest and revealed a great deal about the general dangers of what I came to call (using Erik Erikson's word) "ideological totalism."

Chinese thought reform was impressive in its energies, but neither foolproof nor completely unique. It was related to a number of historical efforts at mind manipulation and drew upon such varied sources as Soviet methods of confession extraction, themselves influenced by practices of the Czarist police and of the Russian Orthodox Church; the traditional Chinese family system with its psychologically minded role playing and related Confucian principles of "rectification"; Judeo-Christian patterns of dogmatic truth and heresy, as systematized especially during the Spanish Inquisition; and certain modern attitudes concerning science as an exclusive source of truth to be imposed on everyone.

I thought it necessary to bring the problem home by examining certain American practices that came all too close to thought reform—for example, McCarthyism then rampant and, to a lesser but still troubling extent, certain educational and training procedures, including some in psychiatry and psychoanalysis. My strong conviction was that we needed to recognize tendencies toward ideological totalism in order to combat them where they existed and do what we could to prevent them from coming into being. In the service of universalizing the issue in that way, I delineated a series of general principles that tended to prevail in a thought-reform–like environment anywhere—those of milieu control, mystical manipulation, the demand for purity, the cult of confession, the sacred science, loading the language, doctrine over person, and the dispensing of existence.

But a number of people in different places could not resist the temptation to embrace these methods for the allegedly noble purposes of their own group. Professionals among them such as Cameron tended to connect these techniques with their visions of *scientism*, their "belief in the omnipotence of scientific knowledge and techniques" (*Oxford English Dictionary*). Never mind that what came to be practiced, as Cameron illustrates, was bad science in the extreme. Because it was "science," it would be the true source of human salvation. It would deliver us from evil, that is, from "Communism."

There are parallels here to patterns I found in the behavior of Nazi doctors on the one hand and of nuclear-weapons designers and strategists on the other. Different as those two historical experiences are from Cameron's experiments, and from each other, they can both be understood in relation to the sequence of historical trauma, ideological cure, and the embrace of a mystical scientism. For the Germans it was the defeat in World War I (on top of previous historical dislocations) and subsequent social and economic demoralization, and then the appeal of Nazism as a revitalizing "cure." That cure included the principle of "scientific racism," with a claim to biological truth so encompassing that the entire Nazi project could be viewed (according to a Nazi doctor I interviewed) as "nothing but applied biology."

In the case of nuclear weapons there was first the enormous trauma *in the United States* in response to Hiroshima (expressions of fear and trembling that were nothing less than a "cultural crisis," according to the historian Paul Boyer), and then the embrace of the very agents of potential annihilation, the weapons themselves, as a source of life-giving and world-preserving power. That ideology of nuclearism led to the extension of the actual scientific and technical achievements associated with the weaponry into the empty scientism of scenarios of "nuclear exchange," replete with "systems theory," elaborate mathematical equations, and the language of physics, while virtually devoid of genuine data.

The original American nuclear-weapons program, the Manhattan Project, was initiated in response to the Nazi threat. The same could be said of Cameron's early interest in mind manipulation. One thinks of the prescient statement on such responses by the French socialist leader Leon Blum: "I tremble at the thought that you are already conquerors in this sense: you have breathed such terror all about that to master you, to prevent the return of your fury, we shall see no other way of fashioning the world save in your image, your laws, the law of Force."

Physicians are especially vulnerable to participation in destructive schemes associated with demigogic political forces. The Nazi doctors were the most extreme example, but there are others. One need only consider the role of certain white physicians in South Africa in falsifying death certificates to help cover up official brutality; of physicians conducting actual torture in Chile, as recently documented by Amnesty International; or of the actions of the idealistic young physician associated with the People's Temple in Guyana who prepared the poison (a mixture of cyanide and Kool-Aid®) for the combined suicide and murder of about 950 people. Physicians retain a certain shamanistic legacy of mysterious power over life and death, which can all too readily be exploited by, or offered to, political zealots.

This may be particularly true of psychiatrists, given the widespread terror of mental illness as well as our professional relationship to definitions of social reality. A prominent example has been the longstanding pattern of Soviet incarceration of political heretics in mental hospitals. Psychiatrists played a particularly destructive role in the Nazi case as well: as active participants in the program of coercive sterilization, mostly of people diagnosed as mentally deficient or psychologically aberrant; and as leaders and implementers of the Nazi "euthanasia" project, which consisted of the murder of more than 100,000 people, mostly mental patients, and provided much of the personnel and equipment for the death camps.

Like Cameron, Nazi psychiatrists made the claim of medical idealism. That claim could even be genuine: the leading medical theorist for coercive sterilization in Nazi Germany was a renowned psychiatrist named Ernst Rudin who believed that the program would help him achieve his professional dream of eliminating mental illness by getting rid of bad genes. And the theoretical basis for the killing of mental patients was provided in a pre-Nazi book written in 1920 by a prominent German psychiatrist, Alfred Hoche, and an equally prominent jurist, Karl Binding, advocating the destruction of those judged, mostly on psychiatric grounds, to be "life unworthy of life." Psychiatrists and other doctors most active in such Nazi programs, then, tended to combine claims of medical justification, political involvement with the Nazi cause, amoral careerism, and ethical and scientific corruptability. That was precisely the combination with Ewen Cameron.

Yet Cameron was in no sense a Nazi. Nor for that matter are those involved in nuclear-weapons designing and strategy. And that makes our problem more difficult, suggesting as it does that highly destructive forms of behavior can arise in democratic settings with the participation of people who see themselves as defenders of freedom or as healers.

We are prone to the belief that, as members of the healing professions, whatever we do is good. But we learn from Nazi doctors, and closer to home from Ewen Cameron, that as physicians and psychiatrists we are capable of our own particular forms of evil. A beginning lesson here is a very simple one: We need always to look carefully at exactly what we are doing, at our precise impact on other human beings, and at our capacity to do harm to others while claiming scientific and professional legitimacy.

There are some who view what Cameron did, and even what the Nazi doctors did, as nothing special, as no more than the logical outcome of patterns of scientific attitude and practice in the modern era. I take issue with this view.

Its kernel of truth can obscure alternative modern tendencies that we can draw upon as well. These include concern for the individual and for fundamental human rights, a capacity for empathy and introspection, and, above all, knowledge of and commitment to genuine healing. Harvey Weinstein's book does much to help us in making the right ethical choices.

Robert Jay Lifton, M.D.

Acknowledgments

The seed was planted in 1985 at a meeting of a group of mental health professionals in Palo Alto. Ten of us have met regularly for several years to talk about writing and to present our poems, prose, and technical papers for criticism. I was to present at the next meeting, but I did not have anything that I wanted to show. The thought appeared out of the blue, and, for the first time, I told my colleagues about a story that I had wanted to write for a very long time. "Try it," they said, "don't be afraid." And so I did.

I am grateful to the Writers' Group for their support and affection. There are so many others who have contributed to this endeavor—the colleagues and patients of Ewen Cameron who graciously gave of their time and emotions; the men and women of the media in the United States and Canada whose questions showed concern and compassion; my colleagues at Stanford University who have understood and provided time to write. To my dear friends Carolyn and Philip Cowan, Robert and Sarah Freedman, and Norman Dishotsky, who read earlier drafts and were kind enough to provide feedback in a way that allowed me to listen, I offer my deepest gratitude. Jim Lorimer, my Canadian publisher, is a wise man. He was the first publisher to call; patient and thoughtful, he waited for me to decide that I could write this story, and then he provided the encouragement that I needed. Curtis Fahey and Catherine Majoribanks, my editors, taught me that a pruned tree can reveal a shape of graceful beauty. To the only two Canadian politicians who have stood fast—Ed Broadbent and Svend Robinson—I express my thanks.

What can I say about Joe Rauh, Jim Turner, and Len Rubenstein? Not only are they wonderful attorneys, but they have been true friends. With Americans like them, the United States Constitution will endure and civil liberties will survive.

The love and warmth provided to me by Rhona Weinstein, my wife, my colleague, and my friend, has carried me through the years. Her faith in me not only has nourished what strength I have, but has allowed it to grow. If I have learned to cherish relationships, and to nurture friendships, it is solely because of her teaching. She provided the glue that allowed me to piece the fragments of my life together in this story. My sons, Jeremy and Joshua, have given me the freedom to work on this book. They have been patient and loving at a time when their own needs have been so great. The joy that they provide, and the fun that they bring, has made life infinitely fulfilling.

Lastly, I acknowledge my debt to Alan Wheelis, who helped me find my way.

Two lives are intertwined in this book—a father and a son. I hope that after reading these chapters, my father will know that he was never alone.

Prologue

One morning in 1979, I was sitting at breakfast over coffee and the newspaper. I do not remember that there was anything special about the day except that my life had seemed to reach an equilibrium. Work, family, community—everything had fallen into place by my thirty-seventh year, and it was good. Then my eye caught the headline of an article buried deep in the inside of the paper and the world became very still. The piece was on the left-hand side, middle of the page. The sun was shining, and there was no sound—a single frame in the film of my life. As I read, I began to sweat and a great pain filled me inside. When I finished reading, I calmly put the paper down and began to cry; the search was over.

The article described the findings revealed in a book titled *The Search for the Manchurian Candidate*, by an investigative writer named John Marks. Using the Freedom of Information Act, he had obtained from the United States government previously secret documents that detailed projects of the Central Intelligence Agency designed to change human behavior. These projects, code-named MKULTRA, included a subproject that had been carried out by Dr. Ewen Cameron at the Allan Memorial Institute of McGill University in Montreal, Canada, from 1957 through 1961. The MKULTRA program was the outgrowth of work that was begun in the 1940s by the predecessors of the CIA and involved the worldwide search for drugs that would expedite interrogation—truth sera. This had evolved into actual attempts to change the ways in which people think and behave—brainwashing. The project in Montreal was one in which psychiatric patients, hospitalized for a variety of different reasons, were subjected to a series of procedures that involved the use of experimental drugs, intensive shock treatments, sensory deprivation, forced sleep for weeks on end, and the use of recorded voices for hours at a time in order to bring about behavior change. These procedures, designed to manufacture new lives for those on whom they were applied, only succeeded in destroying the lives that they had led. For some, these techniques so changed their basic sense of self that what was left appeared unrecognizable to those who loved them.

One of those people was my father.

Part 1: Loss

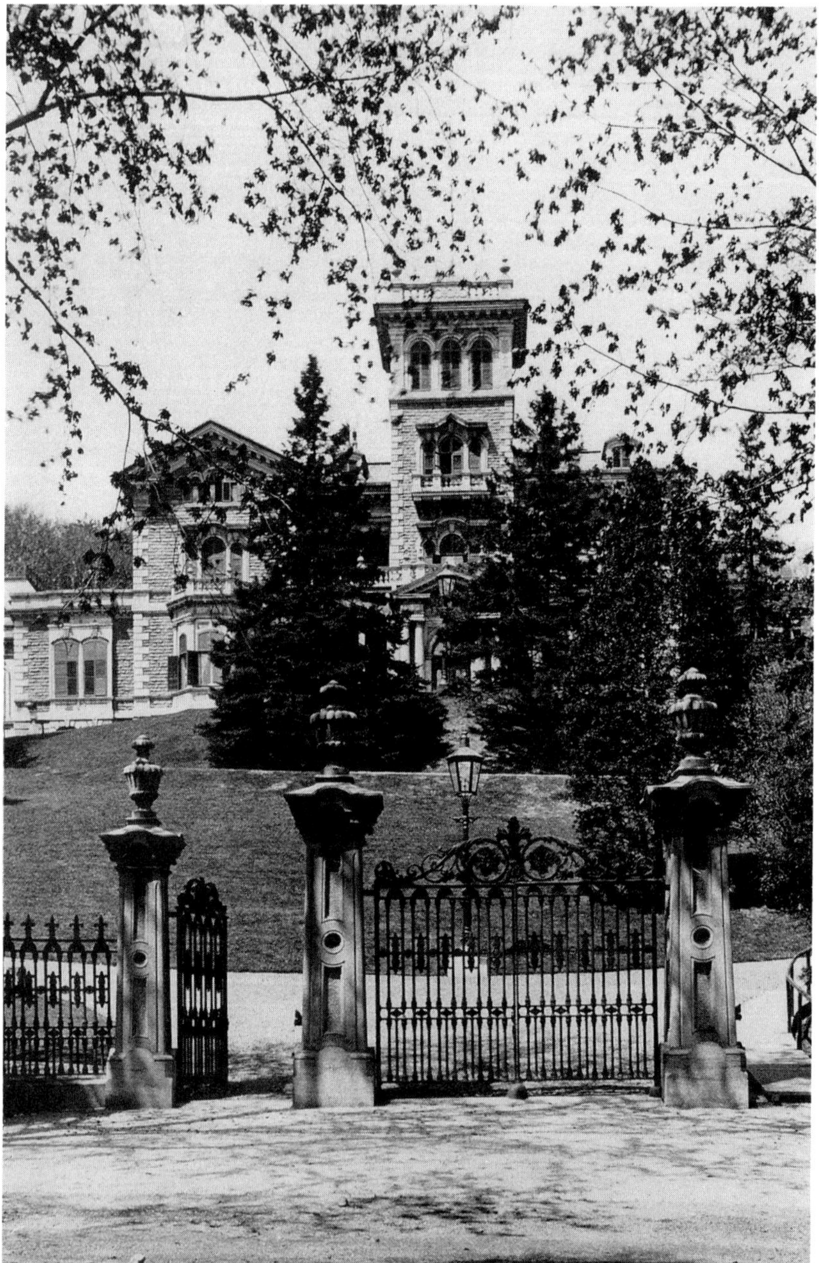

Ravenscrag — The Allan Memorial Institute *(The Montreal Gazette)*.

1

The Nightmare

The first time that I saw Ravenscrag, home of the Allan Memorial Institute, it was raining. I remember that I felt very small as I mounted the steps. The grey stone mansion and the somber skies intensified the empty feeling that I had carried with me for the last sad weeks. I was afraid—this hulking mansion perched on the mountain overlooking Montreal hid my father. I imagined nurses in white, needles, doctors, and crazy people. Suddenly every aspect of my life was in jeopardy. My mother's face was grim as she led me from the taxi to the entrance; she never cried but I could tell that she felt as lost as I did.

A few weeks before, he had been fine—joking, busy, bossing, angry, loving, and loved. Then the pacing began—back and forth, living room to den to dining room—and the aimless walking, the deep breaths, the fear of not being able to breathe. His hand would run over the middle of his chest as if trying to pull air in; his white handkerchief was at his nostrils repeatedly. "There is something blocking my nose," he cried, "I can't get enough air!" I tried to calm him down, trying to involve him in my life, in all that had interested him before. Then he disappeared into that grey stone building that drew to its innards the sad, the frightened, the lonely, and the mad.

I don't want to go in there. I'm scared. What is happening? This doesn't look like a hospital. This is a big house—a castle on the hill—this can't be real. Where is my father? Daddy. . . . Why doesn't Mommy hold my hand? I'm not too big; I'm a little boy. Please don't make me go inside. The plaque on the wall says the Allan Memorial Institute. What will he be like? Please let him be better. . . .

Through the glass doors and up the steps, mother and son, we entered the lobby. I can still feel the cold wet chill of the freezing rain, the bleak late afternoon light, and the sense of being swallowed up by a gray eminence. Inside it was spare. Nothing stands out in memory—a receptionist, a name, and "The nurse will bring him downstairs to see you." My mother looked very tired. I had gotten into the habit of watching her, trying to understand what she was feeling, wanting to respond to her and support her against whatever was robbing her of her smile. We sat down to wait. The images merge. There are shadows and glare from the electric lights; the rain; the gloom; the despair; the foreboding. The door opened and he was brought in. He was being supported; I don't think that he could stand. When he talked, his voice was slow, lower, sleepy. My mother kissed him and said, "Here's Bunny."

"Your son," she explained in a slightly louder voice.

"How's my mother?" he asked.

She'd been dead three years. He didn't know me. My heart was pounding. I wanted to cry. I wanted to run back into the cold winter afternoon and flee down the hill, back to the world, back to the past. I stood there wanting to kiss him, wanting him to disappear. My mother again said, "Here's Bunny!" and pushed me toward him. I kissed him and he blankly muttered something unintelligible. She kept trying to talk with him, telling him about daily life at home and asking him about hospital life. I thought about how I would like to be able to fly, to soar off the top of Mount Royal, out of the hospital and through the tall buildings of the city. Into my head where it was safe.

Months later, I am asleep in my room. The door opens and

a voice speaks. I wake with a scream that won't come out of my throat—just a silent terror-filled nothing as I see the man in the doorway. He lurches toward me and then stops. I still don't know who he is as he turns and I realize that he is starting to urinate. I yell, "Daddy!" He jumps and confusedly staggers around. He is afraid and says, "I'm looking for the bathroom," and leaves. The tears pour out on my pillow. Why am I so afraid of him? He wasn't going to hurt me. I am filled with anger. What is happening to him? Who is he? This is a mistake. Where is my father? Not the first, not the last of a thousand tear-filled nights.

"You can't go," she said.

"Why not? I've been going to camp for seven years. None of my friends will be at home."

She turned away and walked into the kitchen. I followed her and persisted, "It's not fair! I don't want to stay here. Nobody will a hire a fourteen-year-old boy. I'll have nothing to do. Please let me go, please!"

She turned angrily. Her face registered an expression that I had never seen before—bitterness. She seemed about to explode but she controlled herself because she always did.

"We can't afford it."

I started to cry. Although camp was not my favorite place, it was an escape from the daily pain of the last few months. I felt trapped. Hate and anger welled up inside me. I could feel the poison pushing the words from my stomach into my chest, from my chest to my throat, and, finally, the words tumbled out in a torrent of agony. "I hate him! Nothing is the same. You don't care about me any more. All you care about is him." Hateful words spilled out—the rage that boiled inside, the fear and loathing that had grown in the dark months of uncertainty and pain. As the days passed, I realized that my family was gone, and I was truly alone.

I spent the summer of 1956 trying to find a job. At fourteen, I looked twelve at the most. The hours were hot, long, and empty. They were filled with reading and watching my father lie around the house. Toward the end of that first summer, I realized with terror that I too had begun to lie around, waiting for the day to end. I began to wonder for the first time if I too would end my days in a drug-induced fog, as life withered into nothing.

Gradually, new routines were established. My mother went out with her friends to play cards or mah jong two or three afternoons a week. My father slept until midmorning, ate breakfast, and napped. Soon it was lunchtime, and then another nap. Periodically, he would try to return to work, where he would spend most of the day lying on the couch of his office. I went to school and tried to be like everyone else. I became very adept at forgetting what life at home was about, but dreamed still of flying away, of leaving them, of escaping from the apparition that was my father.

"I don't want to go back," he said. "It's not doing me any good. All they do is give me shock treatments and drugs. I hate it. Cameron never talks to me. I can't breathe. I'm afraid that I'm going to die." He was pacing again—moving from one place to the next.

I turned to my mother and whispered, "He's got to go into the hospital again. They're the only ones that can help him." I always felt then that I had to take control. After all, I was the man in the house.

I turned to him and admonished him, "You should be in the hospital. Your doctor will make you feel better. They know what they're doing."

Behind the concern was the dim awareness that I wanted him out—life was a little easier when he was away from the house. My mother agreed that he needed hospitalization; she could not help him to calm down. And so, his family assuring him that this was the best course of action, he returned to the hospital again and again, and each time he came home, he was worse.

My father seemed to have a succession of doctors—resident physicians who were rotating through Dr. Cameron's service at the Allan. None forged any relationship either with my father or the family. My mother tried to talk with Dr. Cameron, my father's doctor, but he gave her little time or attention. A social worker talked to her once or twice, but she was unable to answer any of my mother's questions. No one wanted to talk to me or my married sisters. Once, my mother called the current resident doctor and complained that my father was deteriorating. He informed her that she should not question the treatment, that if she wanted to help her husband she should just encourage him to go along with what they prescribed. His manner was such that she never again tried—after all, what did she know of madness or its treatment? And they were the doctors.

The years passed—two, three, four, five. I can still see the downtown skyscrapers that appeared through the elm trees as we drove up the hill toward Ravenscrag. The images of the changing seasons are seared in my memory. The river beyond sparkles blue as it completes the frame of a city changing and growing through the years. Images of white snow, crystals glistening in the afternoon sun; warm, soft breezes of spring; the vivid reds of maple trees and luminous yellows of autumn leaves drifting over the long driveway. And at the top, that house. Once a place of elegant parties, of the English elite in a French city; now, for us, it was a mansion of despair.

It is 1961, five years after the first hospitalization, and thousands of dollars later. My father has lost his business; we have lost our income; we are forced to sell our house. As I descend the steps from the second floor, two boys pass me. One says to the other, "He's the old. We're the new." My heart starts to pound and a rush of tears comes to my eyes. My rage knows no bounds as I calmly walk to the ground floor. The Hungarian couple are wandering through the rooms. "These arches have to go—too old-fashioned. Those built-in glass cupboards—we certainly don't need all that fanciness."

"*Zaideh*, my grandfather, designed those," I thought. All gone, all that my life has been for eighteen years. This house, my room. The trees that my father and I had planted. Our den—knotty pine, red leather couch, my Coronation coach on the mantel. The family room with its wet bar—my father's pride and joy. Scenes of my Bar Mitzvah. A Sweet Sixteen party, my sisters dancing the lindy and the jitterbug, swooning either to Frank Sinatra or Johnny Ray—"I went walking down by the river. . . ." Tears of Ray's *Little White Cloud*, my tears, my mother's tears, the leaks from the ceiling that we could no longer afford to fix. Mourning for the good memories, for all that might have been; grieving for the pain, for the destruction of a family. We are the old, they are the new. My father was no better, and we were worse.

I stood in front of the open door with sweating palms. When I started down the stairs I had not planned on continuing to the basement. Probably, I had been thinking of doing this for a long time. I shivered and felt both hot and cold. I remember that it was very quiet, almost a roar of no sound, a moment suspended. I had waited a long time for this opportunity; now I would be able to discover what had happened to him. What did I suspect? Maybe nothing, but understanding still eluded me.

It is 1966, and I am a third-year medical student at McGill University. I am doing a psychiatry clerkship at the Allan Memorial Institute—now I, too, am an inmate of Ravenscrag. The attending physician tells me that I am a natural with the middle-aged woman who worries all the time, and whose obsessions and compulsions keep her from living a full or happy life. Yes, I have had a lot of experience in listening to irrationality. But what am I doing in front of this record room? Do I want to know? What do I want to know? What am I afraid of? I feel paralyzed as I freeze in indecision. It would be so simple—just present the request for the file of Lou Weinstein and read it. I turn and go up to the lobby—that room which is burned into the images of my past. Once again, I am defeated. I cannot do it.

1968—one year into my residency in psychiatry at Yale Medical School, and I still have no answers. I have seen a great deal: suicide, psychosis, wild excitement. I have had a knife pulled on me in an elevator. A woman patient has tried to choke me in a meeting. Seminars are interesting but still there are no clues to what happened. I read with a great appetite but leave off hungry. Finally, I think that I have found the answer to the puzzle. It is a late autumn afternoon in 1969, one of those New England autumn days when the light is golden. I am sitting in the office of my therapist—an upstairs room in an old house. Weeks have been spent crying as I have tried to understand who my father was and why I can feel only anger. I am describing once again what I saw and the answer comes loud and clear. He was psychotic; my father was crazy! He had been experiencing a psychotic depression that never resolved. The realization floods me with relief, for I have never before been able to say that to myself. Psychotic—the tears wet my cheeks as I stare out the window at the rooftops of New Haven. So there was nothing I could have done. I wasn't wrong to send him back to the hospital for treatment. My guilt is absolved. Ah, sweet delusion.

And so I became a psychiatrist. The doubts soon returned, but in psychiatry there were still no answers. I was not to learn the truth for another eleven years.

2

The Canadian "Al Jolson"

Sometimes I ask myself if the whole experience would have been less painful if our family had never known any good times. The deterioration of a man, the loss of any family intimacy, the breakdown of all the structures that we erect to support our lives—these images are burnt into my mind, as vibrant today as they were almost thirty years ago. The spotlight illuminates the scenes and the actors as I try to recreate the father I knew.

I could hear him singing as I dropped my books on the table. "Swanee, how I love ya, how I love ya. . . ." It was six o'clock on a February evening—one of the Montreal nights that begins at four o'clock in the afternoon and ends at eight o'clock the following day when the wispy light of dawn reveals Montreal's snow-crisp coat. The long evenings were made for family time, and I was looking forward to Friday dinner with my eldest sister and her husband. "I left my heart in Avalon, long time ago. . . ." The table in the dining room was covered with a white tablecloth, the good silver, and the beginnings of what would be enough food for the entire weekend.

"Where are Fran and Dan?" I asked my mother. "Shouldn't they be here by now?"

"They had to stop by his mother's to pick up something. They'll be here soon. Taste the soup—does it need more salt?"

She was busy at the pots while Marie, the woman who had come to work for us the week I was born, occupied herself by making a salad. The Friday smells still tingle in my nostrils as though my nose has a memory of its own.

"Here, go give Daddy a cracker with chopped egg. He's downstairs."

I didn't have to be told where he was. At that moment he was on his way to California; "California, here I come. . . ." was playing on the record player as I went down to the family room. He was dancing around on the tiled floor, a glass of Seagram's V.O. and water in one hand, and singing with Al Jolson. I liked to watch him. He was so full of vitality and his voice, I thought, was much better than that of the man on the record. Suddenly, he was down on one knee, arms outstretched as he caught sight of me.

"You like it, sonny-boy?"

I started to laugh. He had a way of making me feel so loved, and yet at the same time I somehow knew that he needed me to adore him.

"Sure, here's a snack from upstairs. Frances is going to be late."

He took the cracker and went behind the red leather bar to pour himself another bit of schnapps. I perched on the bar stool and watched as he started on another song.

"You're feeling good," I said.

"Like a million bucks. I always feel good when my children are around."

He was a short man with a belly that somehow never allowed his pants to stay up straight. His thin black moustache and slick hair gave him a dandified appearance which I thought was carefully cultivated. He was full of energy, enthusiastic, and a good salesman. He was constantly performing, selling the good life to his wife, children, and, most of all, to himself. Basically, that was his profession—salesman. He had started out as a "traveller," peddling assorted goods in the small French towns around Montreal. It was a common route for young Jewish immigrant men all over America and Canada, and he had done well. His breezy self-confidence made him equally at home at his posh men's club and in the little stores where he hawked his wares in the patois of French Canada. He started out in business with his brothers, and eventually opened his first dress factory when in his thirties. With some help from my grandfather, he had never looked back.

"My Yiddishe Mamma," he sang. He sang with the inflections of the *shtetl* (the 19th-century Jewish villages of Eastern Europe), "I need her more than ever now. . . ." His voice reminded me of the choir in the synagogue during the High Holidays, and indeed, he had sung in a choir as a youth. I used to try, when no one was at home, to invoke the passion and mournful throatiness that my father could produce so effortlessly. But my voice was thin, and high; I was glad that no one could hear.

"Come and sing with me—let's do Sonny-Boy." I did so eagerly, for this was an old ritual, a cord that held us together through all my memories. It had begun when I was about four years old. We had been going to an old hotel in the Laurentian Mountains, about sixty miles from Montreal. Winter and summer, we would return to the knotty-pine dining room where the owner kept crying, "Everybody wants white meat! What am I supposed to do with the dark?"

The Laurentians were Canada's answer to New York's Borscht belt. The increasingly affluent Jewish community flocked to the hotels where they could play cards, gossip, swim, ski, and pretend that they were a thousand miles from home. At that time, vacations in Florida or Europe were well beyond the realm of possibility. Part of the entertainment was given over to the guests—talent nights and dance contests. Here my father began our father-son act. He would put me on his knee and begin.

"Climb upon my knee. . . ."

"What's my name, Daddy?"

"Sonny-boy."

Schmaltzy, sentimental, yes—but the audience loved it. Forty years later, it is still remembered.

"Lou, Bunny, they're here." Up we went to the front hall where my eldest sister, Frances, and her husband, Dan, were taking off their coats. Warm hugs from cold bodies, a toss-up in the air from my brother-in-law, and my father offering Danny a drink.

"Where's Terri?" my father asked.

"In her room and on the phone," my mother answered.

Terri, my middle sister, was almost fifteen and played the role of Miss Teen Canada to the hilt. Our relationship consisted of teasing, fighting, kicking, and much screaming. She suddenly appeared, in pedal-pushers and a heavy sweater. "I'm here, what's all the commotion?"

My mother and Marie were placing plates of pickled fish on the table with bowls of sweet and sour meat and a freshly baked challah, the traditional egg bread of the Jewish sabbath. Although we never lit candles or said blessings, Friday night was a special time: the dinner was a feast, we ate in the dining room, and the family was always together. My father sat at the head steering the conversation, Danny at his right and I at his left.

"So, Danny. What's new in the dress business?"

Dan was trained as an economist and worked as a representative of the fashion industry, trying to protect it from the ever encroaching foreign imports. My father felt he had a special obligation to prove himself to be smarter than his son-in-law, the family "intellectual," and he tried continuously to do just that.

"Lou, give him a chance to relax." Mother wasn't really listened to, because, in this family, the men's conversation was most important. And yet, it was only because she gave her tacit permission that this segregated conversation could occur.

Often, my father would launch into a discussion of the troubles with the union or with the salesmen from the major department stores. His dress factory was his life. He had built it from nothing; it was all-consuming, and it made him happy.

On Saturday mornings, he would take me in the car down to the factory. Teresa Frocks Ltd.—named after my sister—

was located on the "Main"—St. Lawrence Boulevard. The Main was the dividing line between Montreal's two cultures: east was French, west was English. On and around the Main, the Jewish immigrants from Eastern Europe had grown up. They studied at Mount Royal School and Baron Byng High School and played on the green slopes of Fletcher's Field, the only park for miles. As they grew up, they moved west to Côte des Neiges, Notre Dame de Grace, and the pristine slopes of the English stronghold, Westmount. Many of these men still returned daily to the Main, to the suit factories, coat factories, and dress factories that brought them prosperity.

The building that housed Teresa Frocks stood at the corner of St. Lawrence and St. Viateur Streets. It was an ugly, squat, red-brick leftover from the early years of the industrial revolution. Although renovated, for me it always conjured up 1867 rather than 1955. For my father it was his empire, and as we entered his office he would stride ahead, teeth clenched around his ever-present "Punch Lily" cigar.

"Frank," he would bellow, "Ralph!" My cousin and uncle would come into the office and they would start to look at the newest sample lines. My father would sit behind his desk—a piece of furniture that seemed eight feet long. On top of its vast expanse sat a photograph of my mother and all the children. I would wander out into the factory and talk to anyone who was there. Sometimes, I would take the clothes dummies and, with bolts of cloth, sequins, buttons, and bows, I would design dresses. These I would leave for the ladies that worked during the week as seamstresses, hoping that they would tell my dad that I had great talent and should work for him. Although I have fond memories of the dusty, cavernous rooms, I also remember that I mostly did not want to be there at all, but because it was one of the few times on a weekend that I would see my father, I went. At noon we would leave and return home for lunch. Shortly thereafter, he would disappear—in the summer to play golf and in the winter, cards. Sundays were similar except that in the winter he would spend the morning in a steam room with his many cronies.

"The rummage sale is next week," my mother was telling Frances, "Do you want to help?"

In her early forties, my mother was a buxom, smiling, and warm-hearted woman. She floated through life, enjoying her friends, playing golf and cards, doing some charity work, but mostly taking care of all of us. She was the core of our household. Her reserve came from her parents; none of us knew how she really felt about anyone. She was kind and pleasant to all with nary a mean word, and her patience and stolidity made my irascible and impatient father quite irritated at times. His emotional temperament required a spouse who could calm him and, most of all, create a home where he could come and go—always the travelling salesman.

His travels began in a small town in Romania. The town of Botosani contained a community of Jews who had done quite well during the 19th century. Many were educated and scholars of the Torah and Talmud, and my grandfather, Chaim, spent his days at the *schul* (synagogue), learning and arguing. Rose (Roise, in Yiddish), my grandmother, was at home with her ten children, of which my father was the baby. Certainly not wealthy, perhaps barely comfortable, the family survived like thousands of Jews in the villages of Eastern Europe. Romania had been a relatively safe place for the Jewish people until the pogrom of 1907 put an end to their freedom to be at peace and commune with God.

In the midst of the pogrom, the Weinstein family of Botosani, along with many of their neighbors, fled in the night, heading westward toward the sea. Within an hour, they were filled with panic as the voices of Romanian peasants echoed through the air. My grandmother, Rose, urged them into a deserted farmhouse and they hid in the attic under the eaves, near a small window.

"Quiet, everyone," Yitzhak whispered.

His wife, my grandmother's good friend, began to cry. Her shoulders jerking like a string puppet in the hands of a drunk puppeteer, she could not be calmed.

"Shut up! You will give us away!"

Her husband held her tightly, crooning into her ear, singing a song about a hearth, and children, and the pleasures of learning on a cold winter evening.

Suddenly, a shrill crying broke the stillness. Rose's baby, Lazarus—my father—had awakened and begun to cry. His wailing echoed through the attic room.

"Stop him! They will hear us!" the neighbors shouted, panic on their faces.

"He will be responsible for our deaths. Make him stop!" Yitzhak's wife began once again to sob.

One of the neighbors approached Rose, who was frantically trying to make Lazarus stop wailing. "Give him to me," he ordered.

"What do you want?" She looked up at him with a wild expression, terror in her eyes.

"Before he kills us, I am going to kill him."

"No," she cried frantically, "Give me a minute, I will stop him." As the man reached for my father, she snatched his scarf from his neck and stuffed it into the surprised baby's mouth. To the relief of all, the wailing abruptly stopped. The baby struggled against the gag, but the mother held tightly, allowing him only an occasional breath—just enough to keep him alive. Minutes passed, and the baby struggled to make the air enter his tiny lungs; his hands clawed at his chest in a futile attempt to draw the air in, laying down a memory that would emerge forty-eight years later in a middle-aged man obsessed with the fear of choking to death.

They heard the horses and the shouts pass, and they were free to go. . . .

Sometime in 1908, the family arrived in Halifax, Nova Scotia, aboard a ship called the *Parisienne*. It was no luxury liner; their accommodations were in steerage, in the bowels of the ship. Like thousands of other immigrants from Eastern Europe, they experienced sickness, dark and cramped quarters, and fear on their voyage. Why Canada? The story is murky; perhaps Canadian visas were easier to obtain, or a *landesman* (friend from the village) had settled there previously. In any event, Montreal, with its burgeoning Jewish community, was their destination.

She was a tiny woman, always dressed in black, four feet and eleven inches, grey hair pulled back into a bun. She would reach out a wrinkled, shaky hand to stroke my cheek.

"*Shaine boichick*" (lovely boy).

She spoke only Yiddish, and so my understanding of Bubbe Roise, my father's mother, was always filtered through my mother or father.

It was from her that I first heard the story of their escape from the Romanian pogrom. It was on a Sunday morning and we were visiting her at her daughter's house where she had lived for many years. My father would take my sister Terri and me and we would stand at her chair, or later beside her bed, and she would talk to us in Yiddish. I would smile and pretend to understand. But I felt very far from this little old lady. Her present was her past; my present could not encompass the winter winds of Romania. As we left, my father would take out his wallet and give my aunt a wad of money.

Once I asked him, "Why do you give Auntie Annie so much money every week?"

He looked down at me and smiled, "Because I'm Bubbe's sonny-boy," he said, and he put his hand on my shoulder as we walked down the steps.

After dinner, everyone would follow their own pursuits. Frances and her husband would visit friends, Terri took to her telephone, I would head for the television set, and my parents would go out to play cards with friends. My mother and father led a very active social life with a large group of couples who had been friends for thirty years. Many of the men and women had grown up together in the Jewish area of Montreal. They clung together through bankruptcies, loss of parents, Bar Mitzvahs, and weddings—through the joys of graduation to the sadness of frustrated expectations.

On Thursday and Saturday evenings, they met in groups of eight to ten to have drinks and hors d'oeuvres together. Then off they would go to the temple of Chinese cuisine in Montreal—Ruby Foos. This restaurant loomed like a pagoda of red and gold over parking lots and used car dealerships; it represented to the upwardly mobile Jewish middle class a haven of elegance and good food. My father would enter and walk to the head of the line. With a smile at the head waiter (and more often than not, the transfer of five or ten dollars), he was quickly ushered in to the best table. On his way, he would move from table to table, shaking hands, kissing the women, while my mother walked serenely behind, silently enjoying his ebullience behind her own cool reserve.

I loved to listen to my parents and their friends; they always seemed to live life with passion. They enjoyed each other, they enjoyed their accomplishments, and, most of all, they loved to have a good time. When I entered Ruby Foos with my Dad, I walked tall, hoping that someday I, too, would command the respect and warmth that surrounded my father as he made his way to his seat.

When I remember my parents, I recall their fun. I can still picture their "gang"—newly affluent people in their forties, spending money, perhaps in a vulgar way, but bound together by love, petty jealousies, and the threads that bound them to humble beginnings. I suppose that in a way they were stereotypes; their counterparts were found in Scarsdale, Great Neck, Shaker Heights, the San Fernando Valley, and in all the suburban Jewish villages where the first generation of Eastern European Jews found their pots of gold. Good in business or the professions and narrow-minded in their view of the world, they were assimilated only on the outside—their talk was peppered with Yiddish. My world was secure and I loved them.

It was not always so serene. The sketch that I have drawn hides a darker side as well. My father was a mercurial man—demanding, overbearing at times—and to a little boy, he could be a frightening presence.

I remember one Friday night well. It is dark and I am hiding behind the big armchair in the dining room, the chair that my father always used. I am crying because he has been screaming at me; I cannot remember why but I think that I would not eat what my mother had made for dinner. His face is red, suffused with rage; his voice is loud, hammering at me. I run upstairs to my room and, shaking and sobbing, turn on the radio. Later I creep downstairs and hide behind this chair. My mother, or was it Marie, finds me and brings me a plate of food. The house is quiet, the anger spent. Tomorrow I will go with him to his office.

And so my father, the entertainer, the businessman, the clown, entered his middle years. A moral man, he followed his obligations as son, husband, and father. After years of poverty as a child and adolescent, life was good, a perpetual springtime.

"Though April showers may come your way,
They bring the flowers that bloom in May. . . ."

It was 1956 and the "Canadian Al Jolson" was in his prime.

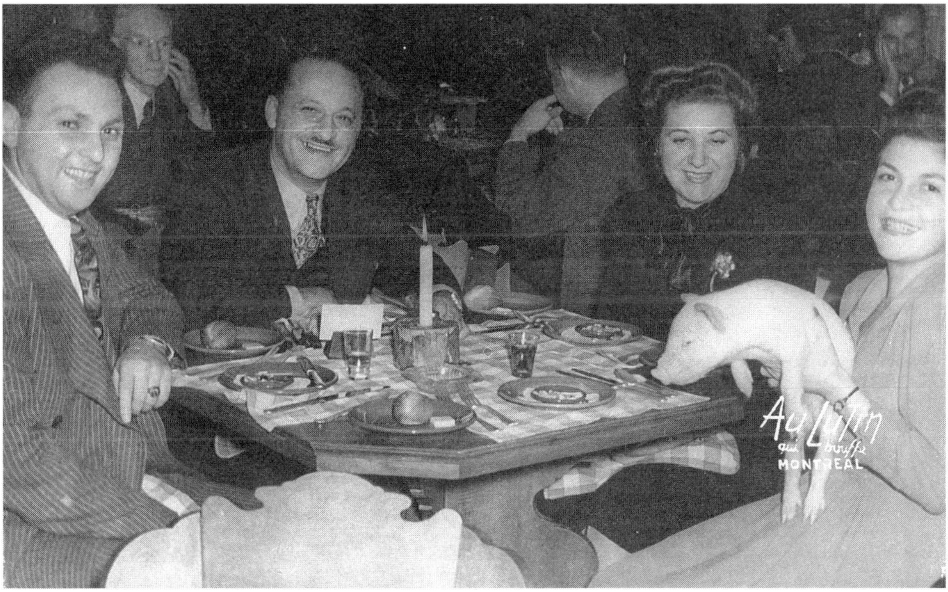

My parents in the late 1940s, at one of their favorite pastimes—dining out at Montreal's Au Lutin Qui Bouffe.

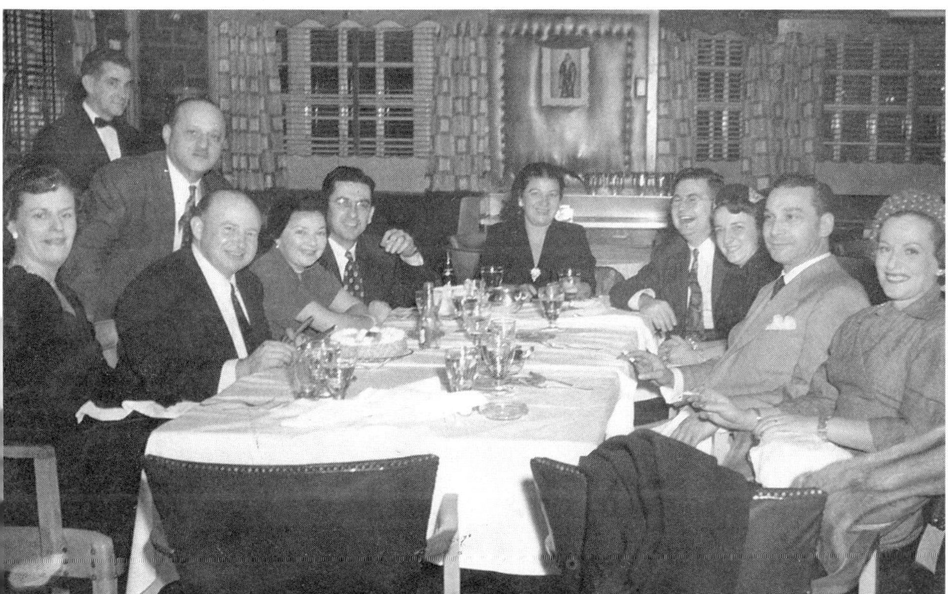

Saturday night at Ruby Foos in the early 1950s. My mother at the head; my father standing at the left. A night out with the "gang."

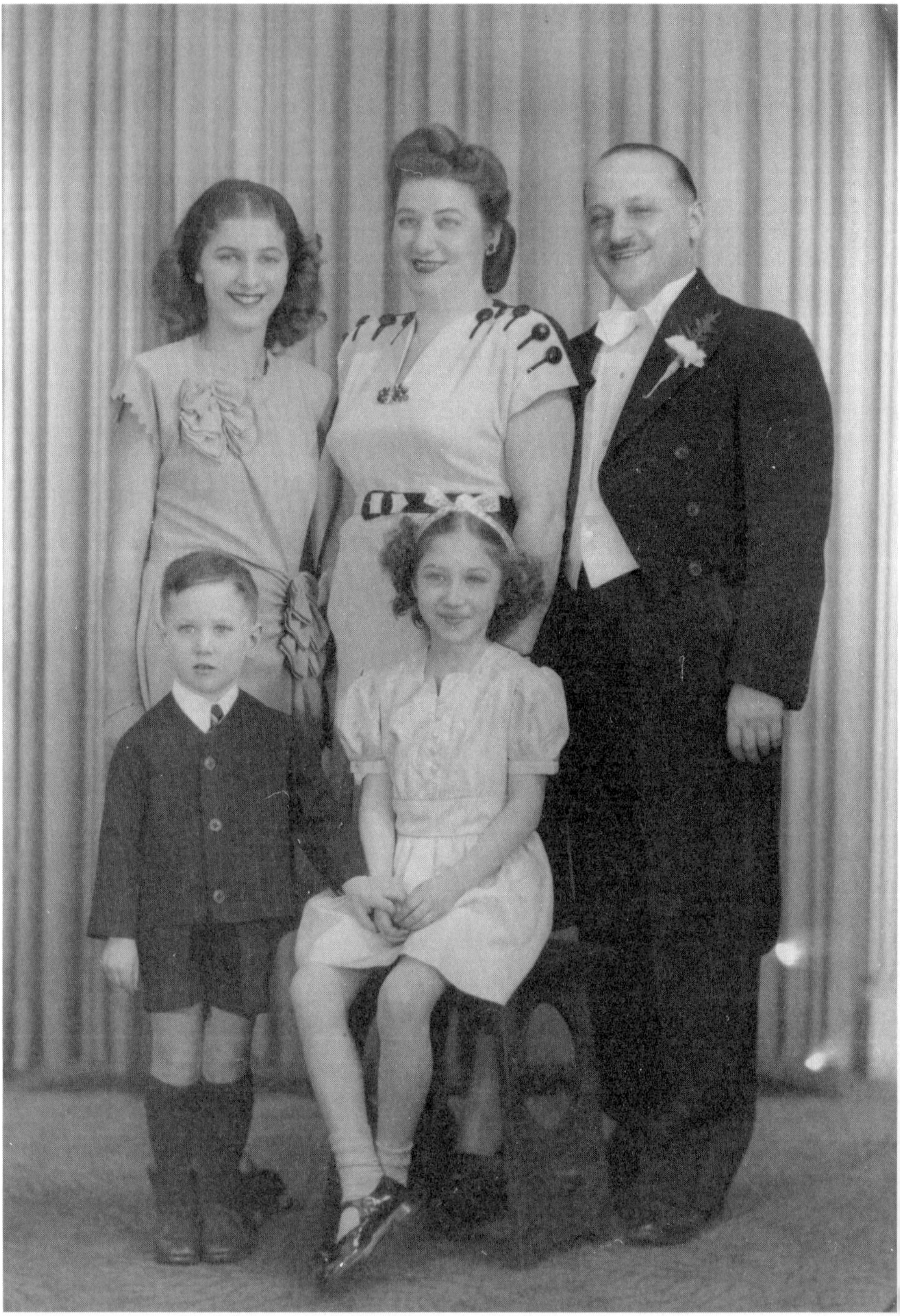

1946—The only family portrait that was ever taken. One can feel my father's pride.

My parents and sister Terri in the early 1950s.

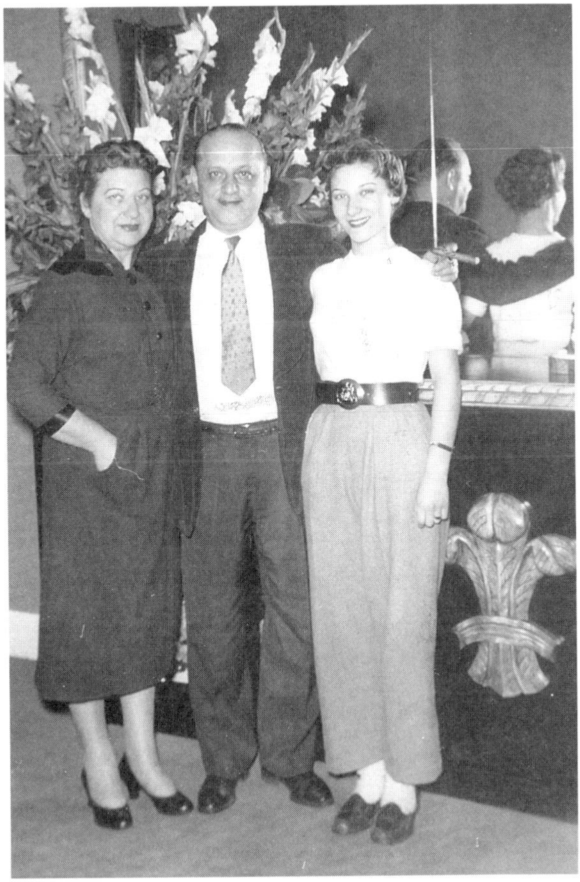

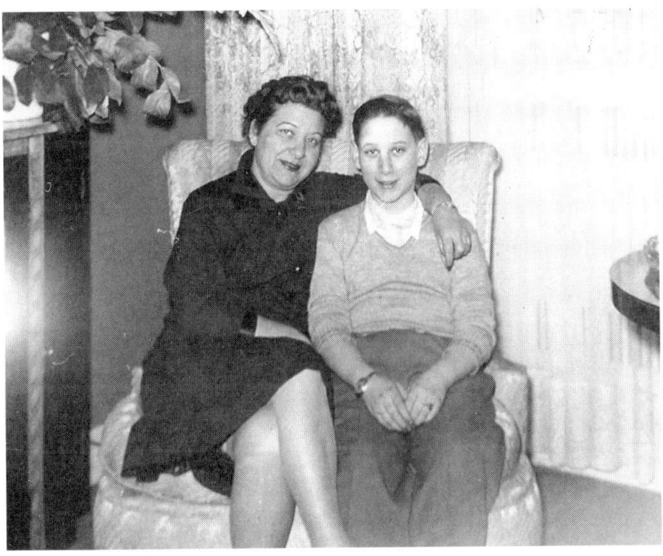

My mother and I in the early 1950s. We were comfortably close.

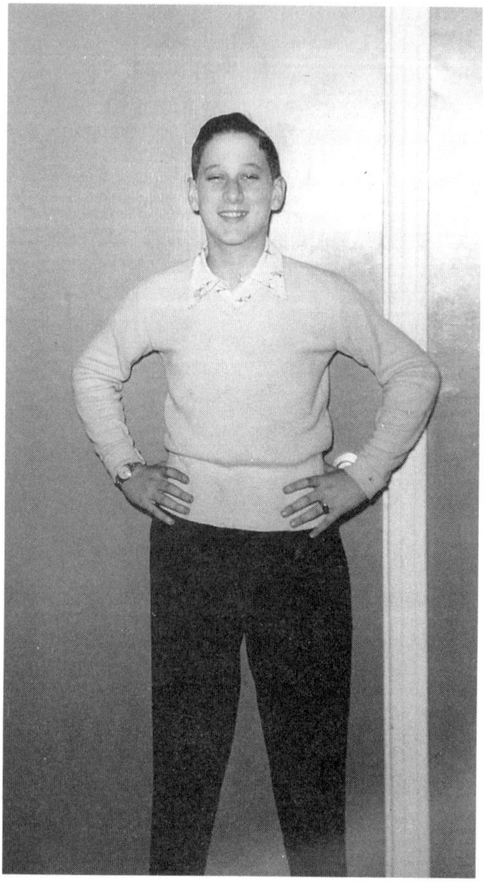

Posing for my sister's new camera, early 1950s.

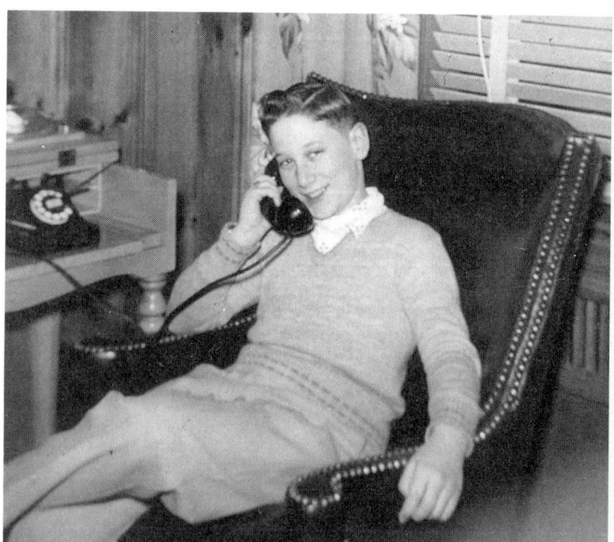

Myself at 12 years old, sitting in our den, and anxious to be a teenager.

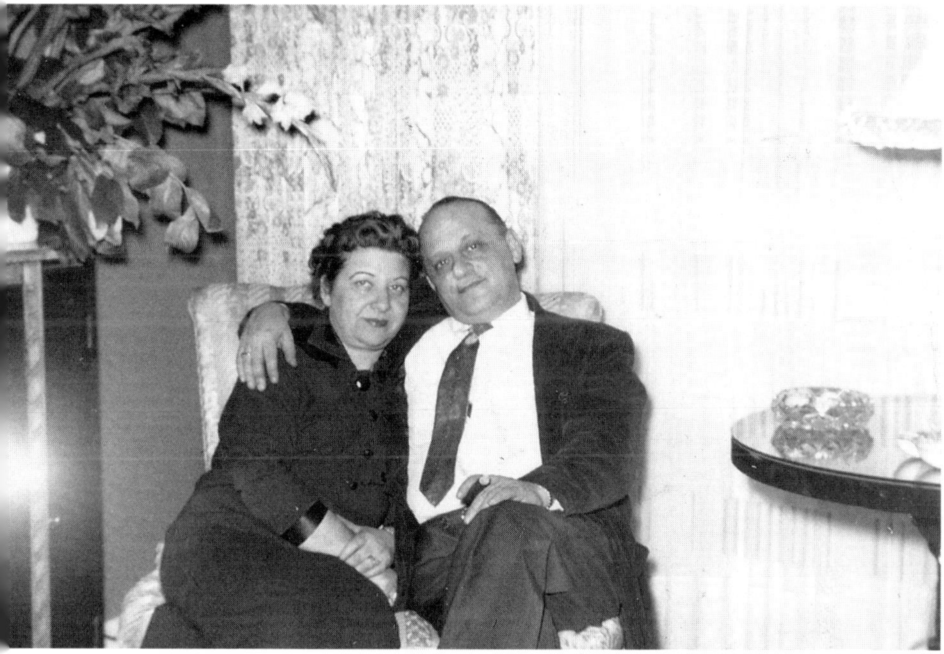

My parents at home in the early 1950s—Dad with his ever-present cigar.

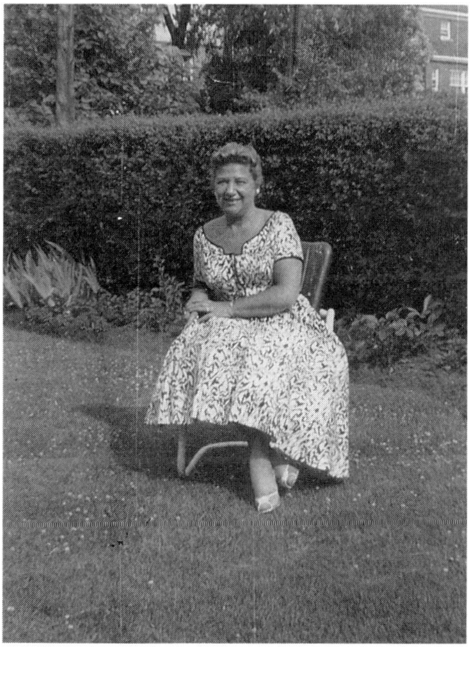

My mother in the garden, dressed up to go out for the evening—early 1950s.

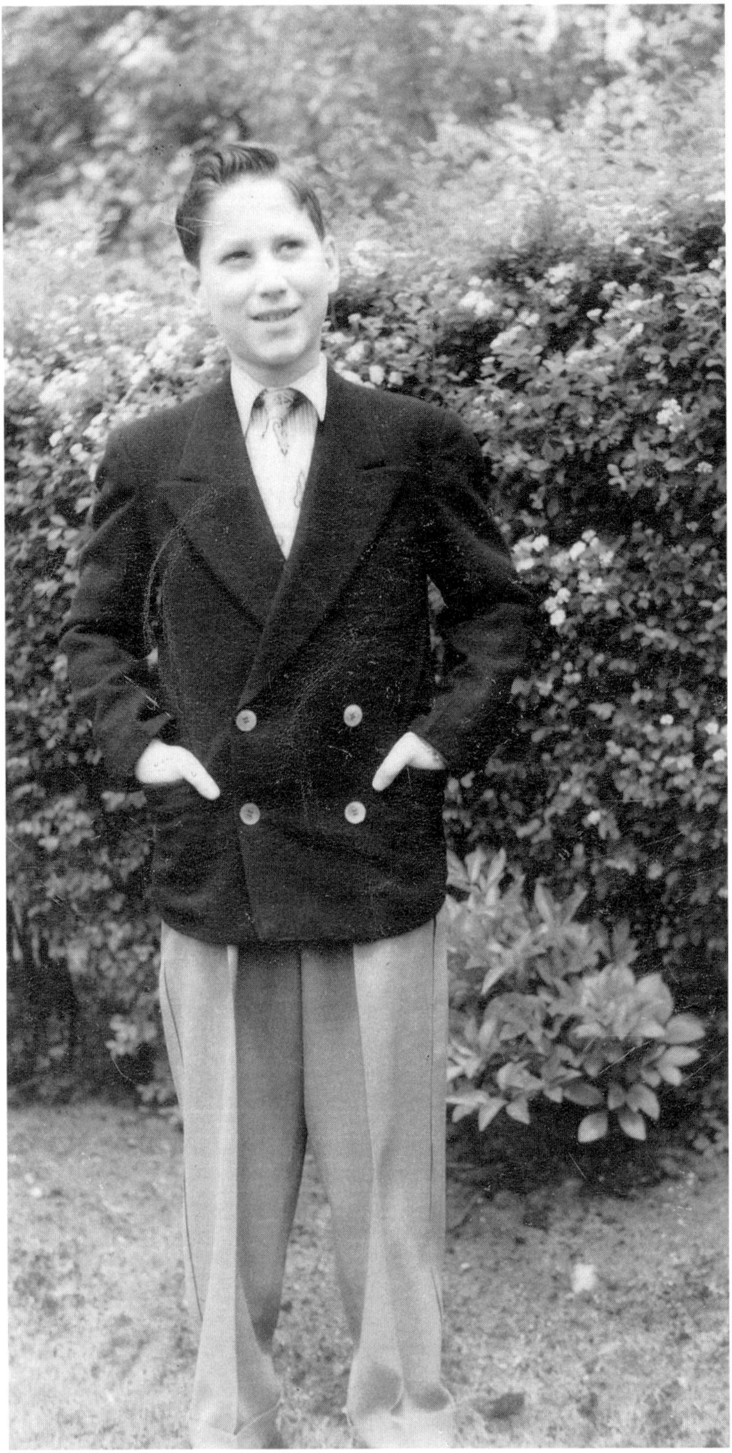

Myself in the early 1950s.

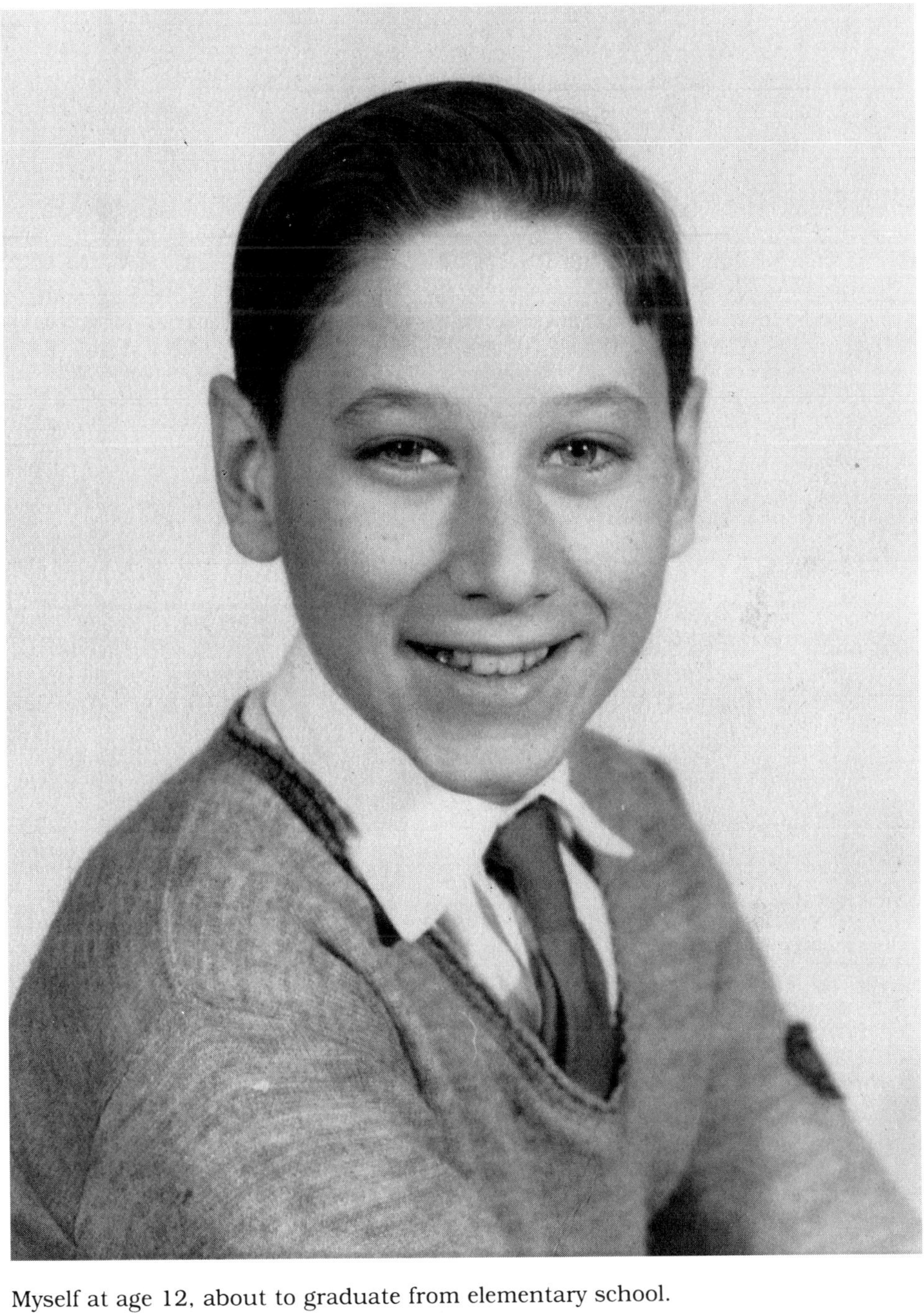

Myself at age 12, about to graduate from elementary school.

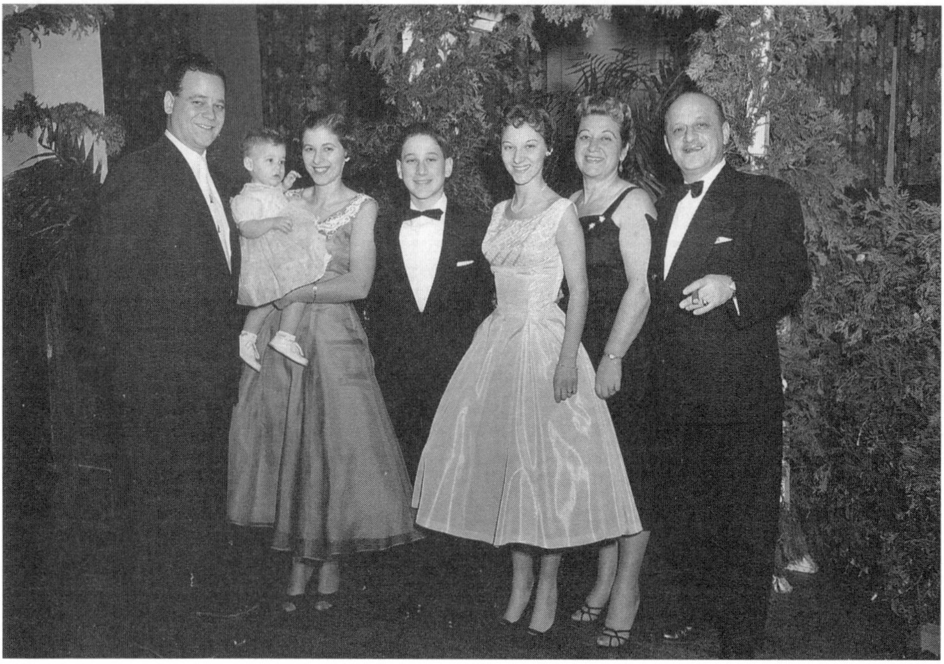

Our family—a picture taken one month before my father (far right) was first hospitalized.

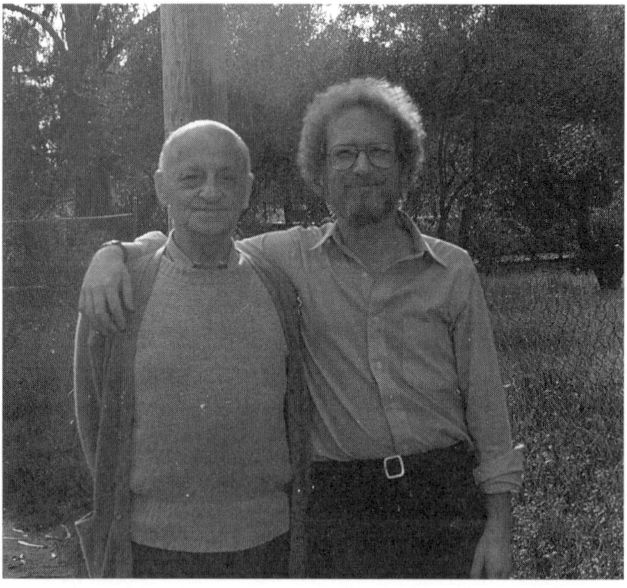

My father and me,
February 1988.

3

Memories of the Beginning

The third child reaps many benefits, especially if he is the only son in a newly middle-class Jewish family in 1942. Not that my two sisters weren't adored, but more was expected of me. I was to carry the family name into the respectability of the professions. I do not think that it really mattered which path I chose as long as it involved university and a white-collar career. To say that I was my father's prize would be a significant understatement. "Only the best for my boy," he would say as he pushed money on me.

By the time of my birth, my parents were in their mid-thirties and had begun the westward trek from the impoverished area around the Main to the four-unit flats or duplexes of the spreading west end of the city. Increasingly affluent, they were in a time of transition as they cast aside the ways of the old country. Primarily, this meant the loss of many of the Jewish rituals that had formed the basis of family life as they grew up. First, they dispensed with the two sets of dishes demanded by the Jewish law of *kashrut* (religious rituals prescribed for the keeping of a kosher household); then the sabbath candles and blessings were gradually allowed to disappear from Friday evening dinner;

eventually, kosher meat was not a necessity, and bacon finally appeared on the breakfast table. Upward striving meant assimilation into the mainstream of Canadian life, and assimilation brought with it the loss of tradition. If *Bubbe* and *Zaideh* wanted to eat with us, they could eat fish or salad, and the word went out—"don't discuss the dishes."

Fitting in, belonging, conforming—the intensity with which my parents pursued this ideal might appear oppressive. They were hungry to succeed. They had grown up in the Old World and were transplanted to North America; money and status would move them into the new world, but they would lose part of their identity in the process.

By the time I was born, my father had founded what was to be his last business. Home was a six-room flat on the first floor of a two-unit building. Ordinary folk living out their lives with few surprises, we were nurtured by a large extended family and the secure repetition of the never-changing cycle of birthdays, anniversaries, holidays, and summer vacations. It is the summer cottages that stand out boldly in my mind: oil-cloth floors, kerosene lamps, and lumpy beds. Each July we would move to Val Morin, Lake Alverna, Shawbridge, or some other small town in the Laurentian Mountains. Always on or near a lake, life was filled with picking blueberries, hiding in fields, learning to swim, and waiting for Friday.

We always shared the cottage with my mother's parents, *Bubbe* and *Zaideh*, so cooking did not fall exclusively to my mother. In the surrounding cottages, many other families—friends of my parents—built a summer neighborhood of cards, fishing, campfires, and warmth. For five days, this *shtetl* was populated by women and children, but on Friday afternoon at five or six, the cars began to arrive from the city. Loaded with salamis, meat, cheese blintzes, bagels, and other goodies from the far-off delicatessens of Montreal, the men made their way to the Jewish colonies nestled in the hills of French Canada. Fifty miles might have been five hundred as the two-lane road snaked through one hamlet after another; past the grey stone French churches; through the grubby village main streets; over the roads where old fat ladies in print dresses sat rocking on wide verandas and waving as the men made their way. As they drove, the noise of the presses, the cutting machines, the fluff of the fur, the chatter of the young French factory women fell behind. Their bodies straightened, the creases smoothed, and, as they drove "up North," the men relaxed in anticipation of their welcome.

Although I clearly recall the arrival of the men, I do not remember that the arrival of my father made a significant difference in my life. Although he was delighted to see me, relaxation primarily involved his friends and the country air. Still, children were an important part of the ambience; we were a significant part of the structure of home. His playtime with us was a brief but tantalizing glimpse of what pleasures life could hold if Daddy were to be involved with us every day. Saturday and Sunday flew by, and early Monday morning, the cars, now carrying only human cargo, departed to the hugs and waves of family pandemonium. A period of emptiness followed. I remember that I would go behind the house and sit alone on a rock at the edge of the woods. There I would dream—and the week would begin.

Probably the two most significant figures in my life other than my parents were *Bubbe* and *Zaideh*. At that time they were in their mid-fifties, but appeared much older. To this day, the memories that I associate with them are full, rich, and brimming with an intensity of feeling that can bring me to tears. This immigrant couple from Galicia was the foundation on which my life was built. Warm, shrewd, ambitious, funny, and powerful, my grandparents, Max and Esther, dominated the family. At times, they were the glue that held the assimilation process together; other times, they could be the force that pushed the family structure to its limits, sending the offspring off to find their fortune just as they had done.

They were in their late teens when the Czar began to draft young Jewish men into the army. My grandfather knew that if he was conscripted he would likely never return to the village. And so they married and ran—first to Czernowitz, where my mother was conceived, and then to Canada, where my grandfather's sister had already settled. My mother was born just a few short months after their arrival. The story is not so different from that of many a Jewish immigrant family and yet, what a gamble! From a small village in Eastern Europe to a country with two new languages to learn; where the snow falls six months a year; where all that is familiar and secure lies four thousand miles away.

Esther was beautiful. The faded, hard-backed photograph shows a young woman with heart-shaped face and almond eyes. Taken in 1906, my grandmother's portrait reveals a woman poised on the brink of life. The photographer captured the serenity and tenacity with which this young foreigner approached her future. When I hold the image in my hands, I recall her forty years after—still serene, radiating a quiet acceptance. Shortly after the photograph was taken, she was cooking over an oil stove, my mother crawling on the kitchen floor as she made dinner. Suddenly, the hair that had been wound onto her head uncoiled and caught fire as the flames from the stove wrapped themselves around her head and upper body. Battling with her hands and towels, she screamed as she fought to put out the fire. The agony was more than she could have imagined, but the struggle continued; when at last she succumbed to the shock, the fire was out. She was left with a burn-ravaged face; one eye remained almost closed; her long neck was creased and contracted with scarring; on one hand, three fingers were gone, and on the other, partial fingers remained, some permanently bent in unnatural positions. To some, the essence of her beauty was destroyed. And yet, I remember her as radiant with great loveliness and warmth; she never lost that special serenity and security.

The comparable photograph of my grandfather is startling in its strength. His generous moustache and slick hair make him look far older than twenty; the steel eyes pierce with firmness and resolve. It is my grandfather that I remember most in the Laurentian Mountains. "Come," he would say, "try to put the worm on the hook." Fearfully, I would try to bait the hook while his gentle voice urged me on. Then again, "Fill your basket with the blueberries. Not enough? Come, I know a special place further up the hill." Sometimes he would return from market with his idea of special treats: black bread smeared with cream cheese and salt, and giant green onions. I can still taste the chewy bread.

And so, in the early years, my life was firmly anchored in my family—a life with no tragedy and few surprises.

In 1946, my parents moved us into the house that they had been building for months. It was a large stone structure with a lovely garden and a view of the dome of St. Joseph's Oratory on the slopes of Mount Royal. The house was clearly the culmination of a dream for my father, a sure sign that he had arrived. It had ten rooms on three floors, and had been designed by my grandfather, a builder, who had also overseen its construction. When I think of the rooms, each holds a store of memories and feelings—the whole being a warehouse of dreams and sorrow. For my father, the comparison with the mean rooms and poverty of his youth provided a measure of reassurance and security. Underneath his dynamic exterior lay a fear that failure could lie just around the corner, that, in an instant, he could be catapulted back to Montreal's east end, there to languish in obscurity. And so the house was a critical symbol to him, and to us, that success was possible and that hard work could pay off handsomely. For him, external trappings were the passport to acceptance, and so he focused on these—going to the right restaurants, belonging to the best golf club, sending his children to the finest camps, ensuring that his wife dressed as elegantly as possible. This need to achieve self-respect by seeking out the admiration of others is a brittle structure because failure, if it indeed comes, is devastating.

It is six o'clock on a warm June evening. School is drawing to a close for another year, and soon I will be on vacation for the summer. I am in my room studying for a test, and as I glance out the window toward the back garden, I see my father stroll out of the house. He is carrying his drink of rye whiskey in one hand and smoking his cigar with the other. This nightly ritual has been a fixture of his life during all the warm months that we have lived in this house. He saunters jauntily over to the porch-swing and places his drink on the table. He then begins to walk around the garden. The lawn is rectangular in shape and bordered on three sides by flower beds—masses of gladioli, marigolds, petunias, zinnias, impatiens, and, my father's favorite, pansies. As I watch, he stoops and snips off a purple and yellow pansy for his lapel. The flower in his collar is another symbol of his status. It comes from his garden in his house; he is a man of property. He turns and looks at the house, and I wonder what he is thinking as a smile crosses his face. Utterly satisfied, he moves to sit, his principal vices in his hands. With orb and scepter, the king reclines.

In many ways, I was another one of his possessions. Expectations were high that I would succeed academically, especially since my father had been forced to leave high school in his final year to help support his family. His father had died suddenly at age fifty-nine during an asthma attack, leaving his wife and ten children without support. Close to the poverty line, the family had struggled to maintain itself. My father had wanted to be a lawyer—"I had the gift of the gab," he would say. For me, there was an implicit assumption that I would become a professional, for although his business had provided well for him, real success was measured by the status of a physician or lawyer. So I studied and won scholarships, even in elementary school, and he was proud.

We never played together; I have no memory of every playing ball or any other game with him. Time spent with him was usually structured around my tagging along with whatever he was doing. Yet there were some special times: every Tuesday or Thursday evening, he would take me to the Black and Orange Bookstore where I could choose three books, and then we would go to the soda fountain at Grey's Drugstore where I would order a vanilla malted. This became a weekly event that was to last for several years. More commonly, time together was spent in meeting his needs. For example, my parents decided to hire a dancing teacher to come to our house weekly. Two couples took the lessons—my parents, and my sister and I. Thus, by age ten, I could cha cha, mambo, tango, and cavort with panache on the dance floor, all of which delighted my father immensely. He could then point proudly to his son and say to his friends, "Isn't he a chip off the old block?"

At the time, I accepted him as he was. I did not question his apparent unwillingness to explore any of my needs. He was so dominant in the family that the rest of us were only extras in a play scripted by, and starring, Lou Weinstein. To see him only as narcissistic, however, would be to do him a disservice because he was very generous, especially to family. My father lived by a very rigid code of ethics and morality. In some respects, this was good; he was a man of utmost honesty and integrity. He felt that family ties were to be honored at all times, and he inculcated in his children a sense of joyous obligation to family members. He helped members of the family financially, and offered the hospitality of his house unstintingly. He loved to throw a good party, and the basement of our house would often be filled with friends dancing, drinking, and eating. He sometimes hired a pianist and singer, a pretty lady named Bunny. Since we shared the same name, I would sit nearby and listen to her sing melodies of the forties and fifties. Often, my father would sing as well and the room would be filled with him, the piano, smoke, laughter, and, most of all, great warmth.

The darker side of my father's integrity was the very rigidity of his standards. He demanded of himself that he always be at an appointment on time and insisted on the same punctuality from others. His anxiety and irritability would increase with each minute any time he was kept waiting. He was unforgiving if someone was less than honest, and he prided himself on his reputation for integrity. He was very conscious of what other people thought of him. He was also a very impatient man. Quick-thinking, he wanted answers right away. He expected and demanded optimum performance both in business and at home; this was, of course, no less than he expected of himself.

It would be impossible for such a man to have no enemies; his irascibility must have wounded some, and I know that there were many times that my mother took the role of peacemaker. She was good at smoothing the ruffled feathers of family members and friends. On the whole, my father needed to be liked, and so his wife would carefully intercede, ensuring that his irritability was never directly expressed to the offending individual.

Lou Weinstein could be a very funny man. His humor tended to be of the Borscht Belt variety, but he was certainly capable of making us laugh.

We are sitting at Ruby Foos—my parents, myself, my sister, and her friend. A rather obese woman enters dressed in a grotesque hat and she sits at the next table.

"Do you want me to go over and ask her to remove the hat?" he asks with twinkling eye.

"No!" we all chorus.

He starts to get out of his chair. "I really think that someone should talk to her about that hat."

"Daddy, you're embarrassing us!" My sister is laughing and at the same time is turning red. Her friend looks incredulous.

Just at that moment, the lady in question begins to laugh at something said by her dinner partner. Unfortunately, the laugh sounds like that of a large lovesick animal hankering after its mate. Uh, oh, I think, we are all going to be undone.

Suddenly, from across the table, a laugh suspiciously like that of the lady of the hat erupts from my father's mouth. I want to sink under the table, but instead I begin to laugh. My sister is laughing so hard that tears come to her eyes; her friend has her fist stuffed in her mouth. My mother, through her smile, is saying, "Lou, stop that."

And then, the chortle from the next table reaches a new crescendo; my father follows, and we are treated to a comic opera aria of Wagnerian soprano and Hebrew cantor blending their melody as the rest of us at the table dissolve, helpless with laughter.

Life with my father was filled with delicious moments like that.

He was a small man, perhaps five feet, five inches tall. He appeared cocky and even arrogant as he strutted around with the omnipresent cigar. One of his great joys was playing cards—pinochle, gin rummy, poker. He had a large group of cronies with whom he played cards in the winter, golf and cards in the summer. He had known many of these men for most of his life, and their friendships were close. I doubt that any of these men knew each other very well in the sense that intimacy was not part of their way of relating to other men. They were buddies; they would help each other out; they had fun together. Much of the socializing took place at the prestigious Montefiore Club. This was a venerable institution for Jewish men with a good dining room, card rooms, and health club. To become a member, one had to have contributed to the life of the Jewish community in Montreal. My father had won two trophies for his work in the Combined Jewish Appeal, and he was very proud of this contribution. Each day, he would go to the "club" for lunch and a round of cards before returning to his office.

In summer, he and my mother played golf at the Elm Ridge Golf Club, also an all-Jewish club, where many of those whom he saw on a daily basis spent the weekends. Elm Ridge was the first Jewish club in Montreal, and represented a response to a markedly segregated society, where there were English clubs, French clubs, Christian clubs, and Jewish clubs. In those years, the wealthy and upwardly mobile Jews belonged to Elm Ridge, a haven for having fun and making business connections.

These affiliations were very important to my father. Not only were they a source of pleasure for the recreation that they provided, but their prestige reaffirmed his success and self-worth. They were further diamonds on his necklace of prosperity. At Elm Ridge, his family could show off their clothes and accomplishments, and he could treat others to drinks or dinner. In this segment of society, the trappings were critical, and my father had learned how to play the game well.

And what of his marriage? My parents were married in 1927, when she was twenty and he was twenty-one. Since my mother had been born in Montreal shortly after her parents had arrived from Eastern Europe, both were basically first generation Canadians growing up in Yiddish-speaking, Old World families. My mother's family was clearly the more successful. My grandfather began his life in Canada by driving a horse and wagon for a brewery company and soon made enough money to buy a run-down house. He fixed it up and sold it at a profit. By continuing to do this, he eventually entered the construction industry, and retired in his forties. My mother had four younger brothers to whom she took a backseat in terms of family influence and position. When she and my father married, they both were working as retail clerks.

Even then, my father needed to impress. He describes one of their earliest dates, when he took her into a delicatessen for a Montreal delicacy, smoked-meat sandwiches. In his desire to show her how successful he was, he ordered eight sandwiches for the two of them! Four were left on the plate when they left the restaurant.

In 1932 their first daughter was born, followed in 1938 by a second daughter. I was born in 1942. My parents' relationship was not characterized by much overt display of emotion on my mother's part. She was, like most of the members of her family, very reserved. She too carried with her the serenity that characterized her mother's personality. This left room for my father's emotional displays, which ranged from pronouncements of great pleasure to temper tantrums. She capably handled him so that family life remained stable and untouched by his extremes. Clearly, he provided an outlet for some of her material desires, since she so readily engaged in the lifestyle that he had set out for them.

To this day, I am not certain what my mother thought about my father. She was so loath to reveal her concerns at any time that none of her children truly understand the nature of their relationship. Subsequent events indicated the depth of her love for him, as she supported and took care of him for the last twenty-five years of her life under conditions of great strain and fear. During the prime of their marriage there were few arguments. Certainly, momentary flare-ups occurred over the stresses of the day, but I was never concerned about the stability of their marriage—divorce was never an issue. For my father, my mother was another decorative jewel. Her good nature made her much loved by her friends and relatives, and so my father could adore her and show her off as another of his successes. For her part, she could vicariously enjoy his ebullience and ambition without compromising her own need for moderation.

I think of the years from 1946 to 1956 as golden ones for our family. My parents were achieving all that they had dreamed, but what of me? As I struggled through my preteen years, I found myself caught in powerfully ambivalent feelings about both of my parents. On the one hand, they could be wonderfully doting and giving people; on the other, they were wrapped up in meeting their own needs. I wanted desperately to be like my father—gregarious and funny, the showman with many friends—but I was also afraid of him. He was an immensely powerful man in many ways, and I concentrated on being everything that he wanted me to be. This compliance made me very shy with my peers and, coupled with the reserve that I had inherited from my mother, meant that I spent much time alone.

Making friends became a focus of anxiety. I could not do well at team sports; baseball and football eluded my recurrent attempts to master their intricacies. My father pushed me to go out and play with the other boys in the neighborhood. I would play until they all went to the schoolyard and the games began. Then I would shrink into myself and feel that I could never belong. And yet, I was not a poor athlete; I was the best swimmer and racer in summer camp; I was an excellent gymnast by the time I was eleven, and I did well in track. Individual sports such as these, however, were not the test of "real boys," and so I was teased unmercifully.

On our family wall at home, my wife has hung a photograph of me taken by my brother-in-law, Dan, at summer camp in Vermont when I was eleven years old. It shows me in shorts, hands jammed into pockets, baseball cap not quite obscuring a face that is filled with pain. My eyes are cast downward, and the world is far away. I vividly remember the moment that photograph was taken. My parents were about to leave after a visitors' weekend at the camp to return to Montreal, about six hours away by car. They had enjoyed themselves tremendously. Since the children of many of their friends attended the same camp, the visitors' weekend was another opportunity for their group to enjoy an outing together. Once again, although certainly they wanted to see me and my sister, I knew that a considerable part of the fun would be the time spent with their crowd. Nonetheless, I looked forward to their visit for the relief it would bring.

That morning, on awakening, my bunk mates had begun to razz me about my inability to hit a baseball. The provocation had escalated considerably when one of the boys had begun to call me a girl. The level of teasing rapidly spiraled upwards and three of the boys attacked me and began to beat me up. It was only the sound of a counselor outside that ended the assault. The photograph does not show the bruises on my chest or upper arms. It does not show the inexpressible longing that I felt, the overwhelming desire to be accepted, and my equally great need to return home with my parents. I felt that they did not want me with them. Summer was their time to play golf, to be with their friends without their son getting in the way. Thus, I was caught—no place for me at camp, no place for me at home. I did not tell my parents what was going on; they thought that I loved camp, and so I preserved their good time and sacrificed my own.

Ironically, I was liked by the counselors. Indeed, I was such an active participant in all facets of camp life that I was awarded the All Around Camper Award that summer. I had learned my lesson well; my function in life was to make my parents, especially my father, proud of me—no matter what the cost. In my zeal to identify with my father, I had overlooked the simple fact that I was different from him. My strengths and interests were not his. He would have to be proud of who I was as an individual—not as a "chip off the old block." Unfortunately, while I had the opportunity to grow up, he never worked through the process of letting go.

Even today, the legacy lives on. I envy my father's friendships, his buddies of the past, knowing that I am often uncomfortable and ill at ease in the company of men. Perhaps if my father had been more approachable, or my mother less reserved, or I less compliant, I, too, would have become more outgoing. And yet, my turning inward was ultimately to protect me from a pain that I could never have imagined that day as I stood before the camera.

For some years, life in the big stone house continued uneventfully. My parents celebrated their twenty-fifth wedding anniversary; my oldest sister married; a grandchild was born. And then, in 1955, I celebrated my Bar Mitzvah.

It was a joyful day. The sun was streaming through the stained glass windows as the choir chanted the liturgy. I remember looking down the long aisle to the back of the synagogue and marveling that all of those people were there to hear me sing. As the Torah was unrolled in front of me, I found it difficult to see; the Hebrew letters blurred, and I felt a sense of rising panic. At that moment, I felt a hand upon my shoulder. It was my father, and for a moment, I felt as though we were the only people in the cavernous sanctuary, maybe even in the world. I lifted my voice to sing, and I entered the world of men—my father at my side. Maybe I even thought that I belonged. A moment of closeness; a touch of intimacy. We were the men in the family and I was happy.

And then my father's greatest fears came to pass—the bubble burst.

During 1955, my father had undergone a cystoscopic examination for kidney stones. He was given an injection just prior to the examination and felt as though he were choking. During the examination, he again panicked, thinking that he might choke. For the next few months there were times when he became afraid that he would choke and be unable to obtain assistance. Basically, he continued to function as before, but toward the end of that year the anxiety increased and he sought the assistance of a psychiatrist. My father was, however, dissatisfied with the psychotherapy that he was offered and sought a second opinion. Lou Weinstein always knew what he liked and what was unacceptable. In this situation, however, his impatience led to a thoroughly inadequate trial of psychotherapy. He was referred for a consultation to Ewen Cameron, professor of psychiatry and director of the Allan Memorial Institute. Once more, my father sought what he thought was the best. And so, in January 1956, my father left the house in the company of my mother; they were leaving for the hospital and the care of Ewen Cameron. On that evening, my childhood ended.

4

When "Al Jolson" Lost His Voice

> I, Mr. Lou Weinstein, hereby consent to and authorize any member of the Attending, and Resident, and Interne Staffs of the Royal Victoria Hospital to perform such examination and treatments (including operation) which may in his or her opinion be necessary, and to hold him or her and his or her associates, as well as the Hospital and its employees, free and harmless from any and all claims for damage or otherwise that I may sustain, or pretend to have sustained as the result of such examination and treatments (including operation).
>
> —*Treatment Authorization, January 1956*

Our family had reached the point of no return. Tragedy, when it struck, demolished all the assumptions upon which the fabric of our lives had been constructed. Exactly one year after my Bar Mitzvah, I stood alone. My father, as I knew him, was gone forever.

During the next five years, new words entered my vocabulary as I was introduced to the world of psychiatric treatment. Shock treatment, including a very powerful form called Page Russell or intensive electroshock therapy, became a familiar part of life. As time went on, I began to hear of other terms: sleep treatment, which involved keeping the patient asleep for weeks; depatterning, a process in which the patient became unable to think, talk, or act in any way like a human being. Lastly, I learned of a process called psychic driving, in which patients listened for weeks on end to recorded "driving messages" or "driving statements" on tape—messages that were supposed to change their ways of thinking and being. Throughout my adolescence, I was dimly aware of these "treatments," but I never really understood what they were about; nor did my mother. In ignorance, we watched as my father was transformed—from man to animal to pitiable creature.

From case history of Lou Weinstein, age 49, Service of Dr. Cameron:

Situation of Complaint: A week before admission, Mr. Weinstein woke up one night with his nose dry. "Then it was like if with each breath I could not get enough air in. I was scared I would choke."

Psychiatric Examination: The patient, however anxious he seemed to find someone to talk to, is never relaxed, and if rapport was quickly established, it was not immediately productive. The patient dresses neatly, and simply enough. His posture is erect and provoking, one could say "Napoleonic." He constantly smokes long cigars. His facial expression is very mobile, showing sometimes anxiety, at other times self-satisfaction. General attitude is very friendly, but in a very compulsive sort of way, and demanding heavily from the staff. Mood is artificially gay, really anxious. . . . Alternately satisfied or dissatisfied he joins in games, etc; but requires to see his doctor at least once a day, even if he has nothing to tell him.

Stream of Mental Activity: Speech is of good quality, logical, but used in an emotional way. He uses questions very often, seeks reassurance. Rate is under pressure, sometimes producing shortness of breath. Tone is whining, all at once anxious and complaining. Main topics show self-preoccupation—"I am the life of the party—I am considered the father of the family, although I am the youngest—I know I am not very patient, I get upset if I have to wait for you—I become nervous when I know that I have to talk to you."

Emotional Reaction: is quite apparent. The patient is upset very easily, spontaneously cries when he talks about his troubles. He gets edgy and shifts to present complaints when a direct question is approached. Certain statements are given with great intensity—"The nurses here treat us so tenderly." The fits of accelerated breathing do not seem to occur at any particular moment.

Clinical Impression: 1. Anxiety hysteria. 2. Conversion symptoms.

Another note describes my father as follows:

> He is aggressive in his manner. There seems to be a strong pressure of thought content. He is very active in his movements and in his stream of thought although he maintains one theme throughout the interview, that of his difficulties in breathing. However, there seems to be a good deal of urgency implied with regard to his symptoms. He gives the impression of being a very demanding and domineering personality. . . ."

The immediate clinical impression was that of an anxiety state coupled with depression, with phobic features. The psychological testing report noted the following:

> The patient is a direct, aggressive and loud-spoken person. He is impatient when questioned and tends to structure the situation in terms of competing with others. Attitude was primarily one of surly compliance and finally submission.

Nothing in any of the admission notes or psychological testing indicates that my father was out of touch with reality; he was not psychotic and not paranoid. The Institute records indicate that his problems were primarily those of acute anxiety. The anxiety was being channeled into physical symptoms that were focused on a fear of choking to death and an inability to breathe.

He was begun on a barbiturate commonly used at the time

to control anxiety. The dosage was rapidly increased so that, within a week, he was receiving 520 mg of sodium amytal a day and 200 mg of chlorpromazine a day. Chlorpromazine is a drug that was introduced in North America during the early 1950s and used almost exclusively in the treatment of schizophrenia (an illness characterized by loss of the ability to test reality). The principal effect of such a combination of drugs would have been heavy sedation.

He was said to receive supportive psychotherapy and was interviewed while under the influence of sodium amytal. After the first such interview, Dr. Cameron noted:

> He showed himself to be just as set as he is in everyday life, boasting a great deal and expressing oversatisfaction with the nursing staff and the staff generally. . . . He is showing considerable urge to leave the hospital . . . based on the fact that under heavy sodium amytal and largactil [the Canadian trade name for chlorpromazine] he feels better; hence we are thinking of putting him on some placebo in order that we may be able to assure [him] that his symptoms are not yet cleared up. . . .

He was sent home that weekend on a pass with placebo medication; the consequences were that his anxiety increased to such an extent that he returned twice to the hospital. Cameron noted: "He is now quite prepared to accept a more extensive hospital stay. . . ." The callous insensitivity of this statement is remarkable. My father would, of course, experience the effects of withdrawal from the abrupt termination of the medications and, consequently, a reinforced sense of helplessness and dependency on the hospital. No concerns were raised about the effects of such a maneuver on the family. On his return to the hospital, my now-panicked father was prescribed a regimen of 680 mg of sodium amytal and 200 mg of chlorpromazine.

By this time, he had undergone three interviews utilizing sodium amytal and Desoxyn (an amphetamine). Dr. Cameron was becoming exasperated that my father was not revealing anything about his past, especially his relationship with his mother.

> We are now going to look into the possibilities of using Desoxyn and the playback, and also the possibilities of using LSD 25 and mescaline as ways of penetrating his defenses. . . . Another possibility for getting through his defenses might be the use of Nitrous Oxide repeatedly since he is a very tense person. We have hitherto avoided doing this because of his concern over choking.

There was no evidence that my father had experienced difficulties with his mother; nevertheless Dr. Cameron appeared to be determined to break down my father's defenses and find the hostility that he expected to be there. This approach was both simplistic and unrealistic, since no attempt had been made to establish a psychotherapeutic relationship with my father.

For the next while, my father was put on and off placebos. He was given several "disinhibiting agents"—drugs that may lower defenses and cause other repressed thoughts, memories, and feelings to be revealed—but "nothing came forth." Striving to conquer my father's resistance, Cameron noted: "Next on the disinhibiting list is LSD, to be given today, 2 ampules intravenously." My father was given LSD on two occasions. "With the first injection, the patient had some temporary hallucinations of seeing coloured Chinese lanterns. He then went to sleep and awoke very agitated and had many fears, which he communicated to others. He felt that he was going to be left and deserted." The second time, on a reduced dose, nothing happened and Cameron's frustration increased because "no new material came out."

The nursing notes throughout this period reveal my father's continual agitation. His complaints about the facility and his need to distance himself from the other patients clearly caused him to be disliked by the staff. The nurses noted that he "spends most of time thinking about himself . . . agitated and sarcastic . . . attention-seeking." These nursing notes reveal a picture of a man chronically anxious, restless, and demanding, with recurring episodes characterized by a fear of choking to death.

On March 5, 1956, six weeks after his first admission to the Allan Memorial, my father was discharged. Surprisingly,

Dr. Cameron noted that my father was "markedly improved," and he was sent home on the same medications that had sustained him in the hospital. It is interesting to note the differing pictures painted by chart notes and patient and family experience. My father attempted a return to normal life, but could only go to work for one or two hours a day. He was on so much medication that he could not function well at work; his business required him to be a salesman, but it was very hard for him to be outgoing and dynamic when all he wanted to do was sleep. Within four weeks, he had experienced a recurrence of all his previous symptoms, and, tearful and anxious, he requested readmission. Both Dr. Cameron and his resident noted that no progress had been made in understanding my father's psyche; the diagnosis remained the same. Cameron's initial notes reveal the escalation in treatment that was at that time being considered:

> We are now planning to explore the possibilities of depatterning and psychic driving with this patient. We are planning now to ask Dr. Malmo to establish some electromyographic constance [*sic*] [a test that measured the functioning of muscle], and see if we can shift these during the process of driving as well as shifting his behavioral pattern. As soon as this is done he should be put onto Page-Russell until depatterning is carried out. In view of the patient's lack of cooperative behavior, however, sleep has already had to be started.

This hospitalization lasted for three months—until June 19, 1956. During this period, for the first time, my father was subjected to the more extreme measures that have been described. By the end of the hospital stay, he had received fifty-four days of continuous sleep in partial sensory isolation and at least twenty-three electroconvulsive treatments (ECTs); psychic driving had begun, and depatterning to a state of complete regression was achieved. He developed bronchopneumonia from the continuous sleep, and his blood pressure was so low that it had to be propped up artificially with medication.

A review of the medical record reveals more clearly how

the process of depatterning–psychic driving was carried out. For the first two weeks, he was kept asleep on the combination of barbiturates and chlorpromazine; at the same time he was given ten ECTs. The plan was to keep him asleep for one month and then begin the driving. The resident notes:

> Last week he was deeply confused, incontinent, and we plan to keep him on sleep for 10 days prior to driving. He has, however, come out of his confusional state rather rapidly. He is beginning to be oriented, and no longer incontinent. We are then reinstituting Page-Russells twice a day until incontinence is reached, which we hope we will be able to accomplish within 48 hours, and will place him on isolation and on driving immediately.

Despite the fact that he shortly developed pneumonia, the ECTs were continued and he was described as "cooperative, though deeply disoriented and out of contact." He appears to have had one shock treatment a day. The sleep therapy was gradually discontinued after forty-four days and psychic driving was started with the patient in isolation. After five days of driving, a note appears:

> There seems to be some question today as to whether or not the patient is hallucinating, which he has never previously done. He looks under the blanket and says such things as—"Come out of there." While looking under the bed he questions—"Are you watching her?" He occasionally startles, brushes his face, makes reference to a dog and a bird. Initially, in the first 48 hours, he responded to the driving in an affirmative way. . . .

Although the file is incomplete, it appears that my father had one week of driving followed by a return to sleep. Some attempts were made to ascertain whether the driving had any effect by observing blood pressure changes. Cameron writes:

> It is noteworthy that the driving did not affect blood pressures which were taken between the 21st and 26th inclusive. It is

> to be noted, however, that we never did have the patient on physiological driving. His memory is quite disturbed and he has great difficulty in remembering things, but we still notice that he has the deep-breathing pattern on occasions, though perhaps not so pronounced as before. He is at present very hostile. The paper which we drove on him is an aggressive one, and we are asking that it should be dictated into the record.

The only record of a driving statement that can be found in the file is a positive one that reads as follows:

> "It is all right to be myself. I am affectionate and warm-hearted. It is good to be affectionate and warm-hearted. I can like myself when I am affectionate and warm-hearted and intimate with people. People like me when I am myself. I don't need to drive myself. People like me as I am."

It is of course ironic that my father had always been seen by family and friends as affectionate and warm-hearted.

Although initially compliant, he became increasingly resistant as the medications for sleep were reduced. His comments became more belligerent: "Is that so? I can't do it." The nurse writes: "Patient resists verbally but does not physically. Says—'I can't stand it.' " After five days, he appeared to be seeing things and responding to stimuli that the nurse could not see or hear. Most of his responses to the voice were nonsensical and irrelevant; however, he appeared to be incorporating some aspects of the message. As the nurse entered the room he said: "Let us get together. Why don't you speak and say hello. . . . well, when is it going to be affectionate. I want to go with you, I know it's important to go with you." But later on he began mocking and shouting back at the voice: "What is that? . . . You don't need to drive yourself. . . . This is being forced on me. . . . You're not supposed to give it away. . . . What are you chasing me for? . . . You're doing that on purpose. . . . Are you trying to make me warm-hearted?" And on another day, "How that I happened to come here? Where am I located here? Explain to me. What is going around? Why won't you talk? What are you going to do? Are you against me or for me? What is this all about?" The verbatim notes indicate that my father's speech could be quite garbled even though he did, at times, appear to respond to the content of the driving tape.

He continued to sleep much of the time and required tube feeding (under sedation) since he could not eat. He lost control of his bowel and bladder on several occasions and was described as "restless, frequently nodding affirmative" as he responded to the voice that he heard on the tape. The nursing notes continue: "Mumbling incoherently. Speech is slurred and thick. Removed goggles and arm cuffs [for sensory isolation] . . . appeared to be listening intently to voice. . . ." During driving, he attempted at times to free himself from the goggles and cuffs, but usually he listened. His description of the experience was that he "saw white" when his eyes were covered; he appeared to appropriate the voice as a companion, so that at one point when the voice was temporarily stopped, he asked, "Where is my voice?"

The sleep treatment was ended after fifty-four days, and my father was maintained on 800 mg a day of chlorpromazine. There appears to have been little change in his symptoms. Cameron continued to push for the psychological origins of his difficulties, and by the end of this hospitalization he had decided that the problem lay in my father's being too dependent on his parents. In examining the file, it is interesting that, although Dr. Cameron did not believe in psychoanalysis, he did use psychoanalytic principles to formulate his understanding of the source of the patient's concerns. Since he was too impatient to use the psychoanalytic methods designed to elicit relevant historical information, his understanding in the case of my father looks like a "leap of faith." It is indeed striking that, not only were there factual errors in Dr. Cameron's understanding of my father's history, but there was also a complete lack of understanding of the life experience of a Jewish immigrant family from Eastern Europe. Cameron appeared to be trying to fit my father into some pat stereotype of personality development based upon pseudo-Freudian jargon that was at great variance with my father's life experience.

By the end of the driving and sleep treatments, my father is described as pacing, demanding, and aggressive, always running after his doctor and requiring a significant amount of reassurance. Ever more helpless and incompetent, he was discharged with the final diagnosis the same as the first: depression occurring in a chronic anxiety state.

As one reviews the medical record, several aspects of the treatment stand out. The treatment given by his doctors was ill-considered at best, and frequently dangerous. No serious attempts were made to intervene in a less invasive manner, such as intensive psychotherapy and mild sedation carried out in the protected hospital environment. Also, my father was being given enormous amounts of medication, and yet no understanding of side effects was demonstrated, and no hypothesis that some of the behavioral symptoms might be caused by the drugs was advanced. The damaging physical effects of prolonged sleep, such as pneumonia and low blood pressure, were ignored. The reports of the driving indicate how preposterous it was to assume that someone who was disoriented, incoherent, and hallucinating could assimilate any suggestions for attitude or behavioral change. The onset of hallucinatory experiences after a few days in sensory isolation had been well documented in the literature by that time, but this did not appear to have been a consideration of my father's doctors. Lastly, the need to break down my father's defenses to elicit the psychological roots of his difficulties is a travesty of the psychotherapeutic process and suggests a therapeutic zeal that borders on the sadistic.

I have two memories of this hospitalization. The telephone rings and I run to answer it.

"Hello." The voice is slow, drowsy, and drawn-out. I say, "Daddy?" My heart is beating fast. There is no response. I wait and say again, "Daddy?"

"Is Mommy there?"

I call out for my mother, and with great relief I hand her the telephone. My heart is filled with confusion and pain. As I go up to my room, I hear my mother saying in a frustrated voice, "Lou, I told you. Your mother died four years ago."

And then, there were the weekends. A pass for my father

meant forty-eight hours of hell for us. We would pick him up on Friday evening and return him to the hospital on Sunday night. That is, if he did not have to go back at least two or three times before then with several telephone calls in between. Friday dinners were now filled with tension and fear as this groggy, whining man dominated the family. Most of the time he would either be sleeping in bed or lying asleep on the red leather couch in his den. When he awoke, it would be to eat or to express fears about his health.

At first, I used to try to argue him out of his worries. This resulted in my becoming increasingly frustrated and angry at him, so finally I gave up and listened. But inside it hurt, and I could do nothing to change the situation. Gone were the walks in the garden; gone were the golf, the friends, the parties. At no time did anyone from the hospital talk to us; no attempts were made to prepare us for his behavior. When he was sent home on placebos (pills that contain no medication), it was the family that had to calm him down and live through his terrors. I am not at all certain what kept our family intact except that my father had left us a legacy—we must always honor each other as he had honored the members of his own family. And so we did.

For the first few months after his release, my father attempted to return to the old life. He still complained about physical problems, including difficulty breathing through his nose, and experienced periodic panic attacks. He continued to be treated as an outpatient at the Allan Memorial and was maintained on two medications—400–500 mg per day of sparine, an antipsychotic drug, and 60 mg up to three times a day of sodium amytal.

In the spring of 1957, about nine months after discharge from the second hospitalization, his anxiety started to increase. He began to worry about his ability to keep the business going, and felt that my mother was becoming more frustrated with him. The resident notes, "By now she has a right to be fed up." ECT was again started at the rate of three times a week. At this point, my mother, who was becoming increasingly desperate, telephoned the resident who had been following my father and questioned whether continued shock treatments were advisable. The resident's written comment in the medical record is informative: "She was told rather firmly that the kind of help that she could supply was in the form of supporting her husband rather than criticizing his attitude or our line of treatment." This was how the Institute helped the family to accept and deal with the devastating effects of my father's illness. During the next week, he was given four ECTs including two Page Russell treatments. After seven ECTs he no longer cared about his business and showed clear memory deficit. Increasingly depressed, he finally entered the hospital, weeping, on April 22, 1957.

"On the day of admission the patient was in a state of acute panic, displaying excitement in the form of restlessness, pacing up and down the waiting room, suddenly stopping, sitting down, and crying." The admitting diagnosis was "depressive reaction, anxiety reaction—chronic." By the second week, he was on 3,200 mg a day of Equanil (an anti-anxiety drug) and Tuinal (a barbiturate), had received his fifteenth ECT, and had begun insulin coma treatments as well. Insulin coma had been developed in 1928 by Manfred Sakel in Vienna, its principal indication being the treatment of severe psychosis. An injection of insulin produced a lowering of the blood sugar and the development of coma. Insulin coma was thought to be useful in the control of excited mental states.

At this time, my father was begun on an experimental antipsychotic medication in conjunction with the ongoing electroconvulsive treatments. There was little change in his condition; he still displayed obsessive preoccupation about his breathing, anxiety, and "uncontrolled" emotion. He continued to complain about "being nervous" and about "tension in his legs" (both of which could have been caused by his drugs). He appears to have had thirteen or fourteen insulin comas and roughly twenty-four ECTs prior to discharge in June 1957. It is interesting that a cranial artery vascular test performed at this time indicated that my father had an "impaired capacity" to tolerate tranquilizing agents such as chlorpromazine and sparine. Whether this was cause or effect is unclear; however, it was recommended that less potent medication be used.

The nursing notes chronicle the habit patterns (or drug side effects) that my father had developed by this third hospitalization. These patterns included pacing, excessive shaking of his legs, picking his nose, and running his hand several times over his chest with a deep breath. He continued to be described as complaining and aggressive, yet he was suffering from the effects of all the treatments. One nurse notes: "Extremely confused but attempts to cover up. Continually asking questions concerning hospital routines, medications, and treatment. Keeps saying he is not getting proper care." At discharge, there was no change in the broken man that he had become.

I have recently come across a short story that I wrote in 1959 when I was seventeen years old. I remember sitting at the desk wrapped up in the tale of a boy who had lost his father. The room was dark except for the small table lamp, and I worked with a feverish intensity for three hours. When I reached the end, I was overcome with sadness—an ache that makes sense to me only as I look back in time. Some twenty-five years later, I can see the tale as a metaphor for the pain that permeated my life. I titled it "Out of the Darkness" and it was supposed to be a sequel to a Faulkner story that we had read in class. Tom was a fourteen-year-old Southern boy whose father had been killed in an automobile accident two years previously. His brother had gone off to the southern Pacific to fight the Japanese during World War II, and the story focuses on the relationship between the boy, who has had to shoulder the responsibilities of manhood long before his time, and his mother. Tom waits anxiously for letters from his brother as he struggles to keep the farm together. One day, a telegram arrives with the news that his brother is missing in action:

> Mrs. Grier moaned, "Oh no, not my boy," and then she wept uncontrollably. Tom shook his head; this could not be true, not Peter, not Peter Grier. Then he was in his mother's arms, and sorrow flooded their hearts as it did the hearts of many that night.
>
> Thomas Grier was bitter then, and his bitterness grew. His

> simple heart could not grasp the cause that took his brother from him and his mother. Why? He asked that question a hundred times, a thousand—why? He could not understand why God had done this, and Tom Grier cried, until he could cry no more.
>
> August came, and September, and with September came the news, the Japanese had surrendered. The world went mad with joy, the war was over! In the Grier house, however, melancholy reigned. Tom did not care about the war; he only knew that Pete would not be coming home with the rest. What had once been a beautiful world to him was now devoid of all that was beautiful and good.

The story has a happy ending because a month later, as Tom drags himself through another day, he sees a familiar figure on the road:

> Could it be? Was it possible? The answer came to him in a flash—yes, it can be. It is! Tom began to run faster and faster. The tears streamed down his face as he shouted, "Pete! Pete!" His brother had come home.

I finished the last word and I put my head down on the desk. I remember that I felt unutterably alone. The enormity of the emptiness filled me with despair, but I never made the connection between the story and my life. This adolescent tale, complete with happy ending, was published in my high school yearbook. My social self accepted the accolades; that night, I could not eat dinner.

For the next three and a half years, my father was treated by Dr. Cameron both in the Allan Memorial's day hospital and as an outpatient. After discharge, he was maintained on the experimental drug and electroconvulsive treatments on a weekly or biweekly basis. In addition to his usual symptoms, he was sleepy all the time and consequently unable to do more than go to work and sleep on the office couch. The notes reveal that visits with Cameron were focused on monitoring symptoms and drug response. As usual, there seemed to be little understanding of how little my father was capable of functioning: "he is working steadily in the office," his file says. In addition, he began to experience neurological side effects of the medication: "he complains as usual about minor things, for instance his wrist jerks on occasion and sometimes his leg[,] which seems to be no more than a muscular jerk or twitch." Gradually, over the next year and a half, he began to complain less of the breathing problem and nervousness, but he was so sedated that his ability to participate in life was severely limited.

Ultimately, because of increased shaking of his leg and "anxiety," he was begun once more on sleep treatments. These were carried out in the day hospital and lasted for several hours at a time. Whether his pacing and leg shaking were attributable to the experimental drug does not seem to have been a consideration; rather, this was seen as an exacerbation of his condition, and the treatment escalated once again. During one ECT he lost a tooth while experiencing a convulsion; during another sleep treatment, following an injection of Pentothal, "he had something of a collapse and took some time to re-establish his circulation again." How this loss of oxygen to the brain affected him is not clear since so much else was taking place at the time. The shock treatments appear to have been stopped after seventy ECTs, but there is no statement in the chart as to why that decision was made. On a monthly basis, therefore, he continued with the sleep treatment and occasional other drugs.

In 1961, he was forced to give up his business. The warning signs had been present for a long time. Although there were many employees, a manager, and salesmen, the factory was basically a one-man affair, particularly in the area of sales. Since my father could no longer meet with the buyers from the major department stores, business was going elsewhere. And since other family members were involved in the business, pressure had begun to mount for the now unprofitable business to be sold. This is one of the few times that I remember quarrels and anger between my parents. My father's entire life and his sense of self was wrapped up in Teresa Frocks; selling the factory represented for him the end of the road. He would no longer have the success that had given him status in his family and with his friends. My brother-in-law tried to intervene on my father's behalf, but my mother could not fight with the other members of the family.

There being no direct offer for the business, it was auctioned off in bits and pieces and brought in less than half of what it was worth. Shortly thereafter, it was discovered that the company's losses were, to a large extent, attributable to the bookkeeper, who had embezzled thousands of dollars. Since my father was incapable of monitoring the finances of the company, and since no one else had the capacity to do so, the bookkeeper made off with the money and disappeared.

With the demise of Teresa Frocks, the ambitious, power-oriented showman lost any remaining zest for life. Like a wounded animal, he curled up in his bed, weeping and gasping for breath. His greatest fears had been realized; he could no longer stand up as a man. More was to come, because soon my mother came to the realization that we could not afford to keep up the house. I was, by that time, nineteen and a sophomore pre-med student at McGill University. Given her fears of financial ruin, I supported her in the decision to sell the house, and helped her to find a small apartment. We did not ask my father's opinion, nor did he participate in choosing his next home. I had begun to see him as the rest of the world did—weak, ineffectual, a drain on all of us, and a pathetic creature. As the time came for us to move, the strain began to wreak havoc on my ability to study. I could not concentrate on organic chemistry or quantitative analysis; my ability to lead a life that excluded the fact of my father's illness was increasingly compromised. A scholarship student in my freshman year, I scraped through the second year and seriously compromised my chances for medical school. Life was closing in for all of us—my father, my mother, and myself. Both sisters had married by 1957 and left the house: the pressure of dealing with my parents fell fully on me.

I don't know how I got through my adolescence. My life experience was so different from that of my friends that I could not share with them the fears and sadness that haunted my daily existence. My brother-in-law Danny became my sole source of support during those years. I would run to Danny and Frances's house as often as I could to escape the smothering atmosphere of my home. At one point, when I was fifteen or sixteen, Danny offered to take me into their family; he even said that if my parents refused, he would take it to court. I was confused. Part of me longed for escape; more of me felt that I could not abandon my parents. I had lost sight of any goals or desires that I could call my own.

It is a warm June day. My parents and I have driven over to my sister's house to visit—a trip that is harrowing because my father insists on driving. Despite the medication and slow reflexes, he cannot be talked out of taking the wheel. I sit on the edge of the backseat, warning him about driving in the middle of the road, reminding him to stop at the light. He is irritated with me as he rolls along at fifteen miles an hour. My mother tries to intervene but her loyalties are torn and she cannot do other than attempt to mediate. I know that she too is afraid of his driving. By the time we arrive at my sister's front door, I am distraught, my mother is withdrawn, and my father is oblivious.

We enter the house and the strain is obvious. Frances and Danny try to put us all at ease. When the grandchildren come out, my mother immediately turns to them while my father takes to the couch, ready to fall asleep. Alone. I feel alone. The people in the room drift farther and farther away.

My father is snoring; my mother is laughing with her eldest granddaughter; my sister is talking to her. Danny looks over at me. He sees me in pain and asks me to come outside with him. I feel as though I am going to explode; the world is closing in. Who are these people? Where are my parents? I am trapped.

I jump out of my chair and bolt from the room. Outside, the world is filled with warmth, but I feel nothing as I run down the street. Dimly, I am aware of my brother-in-law behind me. He grabs me as we reach the corner. I dissolve in tears as he holds me.

"I can't go on. I'm suffocating at home. I can't live with them. Help me. . . ."

He did. With words, unstinting kindness, and love, Danny saved my life in a thousand ways. Without his affection, I would never have survived.

By the autumn of 1961, my father had lost his livelihood and his home—no more pansies; no more basement bar; no more Friday dinners in the dining room. Cameron's only comment: "He has unfortunately given up his business, because he felt he could not attend to it, and he is lying around doing relatively little. He is to have another treatment and should return in a month." Through all of these years, many thousands of dollars had been spent by my parents for the medical care that my father had received from Dr. Cameron and the Allan Memorial—health insurance had covered only the first hospitalization. With the medical expenses and a significant loss of income, the family was squeezed financially. To further compound the blows to my father's self-esteem, he was forced to borrow money from other family members.

It was then that my relationship to my revered grandparents began to change. From kindly *Bubbe* and *Zaideh*, they became the principal source of funds that allowed my parents to survive. What had been done out of love gradually took on for me a sense of moral obligation. Acts of kindness became interpreted in my mind as debts to be repaid. With growing ambivalence, I realized that another of my sources of strength had become contaminated by the insidious decline of my father. Bonds of love and respect coalesced into a web of shame and sorrow.

Every Sunday, from the time that I was at least five years old, my mother, my sister, and I had spent the afternoon at my grandparents' house. Eventually, only my mother and I still visited. When I close my eyes, I can picture a room with high ceilings, oriental rug on the floor, photographs of children and grandchildren, and two special joys: a console radio from the 1930s that received shortwave stations, and a very early Victrola with RCA records from a time long before I was born. The snow would be falling, the wind howling. Inside, *Bubbe*, *Zaideh*, and my mother would be chatting in Yiddish while I vainly tried to follow the conversation. In their front room stood a dark walnut sentinel, a massive grandfather clock that regularly timed for me the passage of the long afternoon. Every one of the grandchildren and great-grandchildren who visited during those years has a vivid memory of the clock. It dominated the house and symbolized for me the continuity of the family. Where had it come from? Through what joys and sadnesses had it chimed? Would it continue to watch over us as we grew?

At three o'clock, *Zaideh* called us in to tea. Crackers and strawberry jam, *Bubbe*'s cookies, fruit, and strong tea—even for me. Usually at five, my father would call. We would either go down to his club to meet him for dinner, or some other arrangement would be made for Sunday dinner, and the day would draw to its close.

For years, these afternoons were an oasis of peace. Never have I felt as secure and content as I did during those winter Sundays. But with the advent of my father's illness and my parents' increasing dependence on *Bubbe* and *Zaideh* for funds, the afternoons became filled with bitterness. Somehow my mother was different with them, perhaps even obsequious. They seemed to feel that they had more right to advise her in decision making. Before my eyes, she was turning into a dutiful daughter of sixteen. It became increasingly difficult for me to spend my Sundays at their home, but I continued to go for her, for my mother, almost through the end of high school.

In December 1961, faced with mounting losses, my father's condition began to deteriorate and his anxiety increased. He was then readmitted to the hospital with the same diagnosis as previously, "severe neurotic anxiety with conversion symptoms." Conversion symptoms refer to physical complaints that result from emotional conflict. The patient is thought to express emotional pain through disturbances in the functioning of the body.

He was initially given another experimental medication, but, after a week, sleep treatment was again started. This version of the treatment was designed to keep him asleep every second day under the influence of barbiturates and chlorpromazine. On the alternate days, he was given lesser dosages of the medications. Toward the end of the first month, a decision was made to begin psychic driving once again. Cameron and his group were now more sophisticated in their practices and were trying to develop ways to determine whether the driving was effective. A nurse's note records that films were taken of my father so that his movements could be assessed before and after the procedure. Following twenty days of semi-sleep, he was begun on a positive driving procedure. The driving statement was as follows: "You feel friendly towards people. You like to feel intimate with others. You can get along with people by being yourself. You feel neat and tidy. If you see paper on the floor, you pick it up." The second to last statement was in response to my father's loss of a sense of personal cleanliness and neatness. The last statement reflected an effort to see if driving would in fact produce a concrete behavioral change that was directly observable.

A nurse noted my father's response to the semi-sleep and driving: "It gets rather lonely lying here all day listening to the same thing over and over again." The nurse also commented: " . . . doesn't think it has given him any confidence in himself as a person or helped him in society. . . ." Dr. Cameron saw him as "apathetic" and "lacking in interest or drive"—he appeared to be burned-out. Prior to discharge on February 27, 1962, he had received at least twenty-six days of semi-sleep and eighteen days of driving. He was discharged to the day hospital to continue both the sleep treatment and driving. This continued for another four months, after which time he requested that the treatment regimen be discontinued. He was transferred to the outpatient clinic. An unsigned note in the clinic's records is quite revealing:

> This is a new patient who was recently discharged from Day Hospital West. He is an extremely difficult case to work with. He has gone downhill so that he is almost completely apathetic at the present time. No satisfactory explanation or diagnosis for his condition has really been offered at present. He is on driving and sedative medication as well as occasional treatments.

Over the following ten months, my father was given barbiturates and chlorpromazine, and was afraid to go out of the house. He was seen on an irregular basis, primarily for prescription refills, and by April 1963, a particularly illuminating note by a clinic resident makes the following observation: "As usual he failed to come to his appointment, and no doubt will turn up one of these days for a new prescription. I have a feeling that he is becoming addicted to his drugs." This was the first acknowledgment that the treatment itself might be problematic. The same resident noted shortly thereafter that my father was himself attempting to reduce his medications but says: "Unfortunately we will have to put up with this patient, although it is disturbing to recognize that we are doing nothing for him apart from creating a pill addict. At the present moment there seems to be no other possibility."

By 1964, my father had begun to wean himself away from the Allan Memorial, although he continued to go there sporadically for some years. He remained on the antipsychotic medication, but at a markedly reduced dose. The last entry in his file is from September 1970 and indicates no contact since May of that year. The note ends: "other arrangements should be made if he returns." Although there are missing parts of the record, it does not appear that my father was seen by Dr. Cameron following the hospitalization of 1961. Perhaps this was due to my father's inability to pay, or perhaps there was some other reason. My father does not remember. What he can recall is that he no longer wanted to have anything to do with the Allan Memorial Institute.

My father was left with severe disabilities. He lost all sense of personal cleanliness or awareness of others. He developed a habit of constantly humming, especially at mealtimes, and this made sitting with him almost unbearable. His life revolved around a series of rituals that had to be followed each day without exception. His thinking was very rigid and concrete, and his conversation with others was limited. He sustained extensive but patchy memory loss for most of the years from 1955 through 1964. Episodes of anxiety decreased but were replaced by periods of depression and apathy. The "Canadian Al Jolson" was no more.

Through all of this, my mother stood by, cajoling him, making sure he stayed clean, trying to interest him in some kind of social life. Intimacy was impossible and companionship nonexistent—I do not know what sustained her.

As for me, throughout the early 1960s I continued to try to escape. In 1960, I took all the money that I had and went on a Youth Hostel bicycle trip to Europe for three months. During those weeks I was another person and felt freer than I ever had. I took the opportunity to write a letter to my father, telling him how very much I loved him—from three thousand miles away I could not escape the guilt. And yet those weeks crystallized for me the possibility that I could define myself as a person apart from my family. In retrospect, the exhilarating taste of carefree existence, coming, as it did, four years into my father's decline, provided me with hope. I returned to Montreal filled with enthusiasm, but my joy was quickly dashed by my father's rehospitalization, the end of his business, and the loss of our house. And so it went, up and down through my late adolescence.

Two facets of my character were particularly honed during those years. The first was my continued inability to feel comfortable with peers. On the outside, I appeared to fit in well. I was a member of a fraternity and my college friendships had developed through that organization, yet none of my friends could have had a shred of understanding about the life I returned to when I came home at night. So I was removed. Secondly, I had become so terrified of intimacy that my relationships with women could progress only so far, and then I needed to withdraw. I became known for my September to April relationships. Each year of university, I became enamored of a new woman; I would romance her, enjoy her company, and develop a measured amount of closeness. As soon as she began to desire more, I would feel myself withdraw, and before she could understand that anything was amiss, I would terminate the friendship abruptly. Once again, I knew how to play the game. On the outside, I appeared successful—academically and socially. Within, I lived in despair; I mourned for what had been; I searched to understand what was; and I shared with no one.

I graduated from McGill University with a Bachelor of Science degree in 1963, and later that year entered McGill's medical school. I continued to deal with the pressures at home, but, by my early twenties, the loneliness had become increasingly hard to bear. As I studied to become a physician, I knew that I had to find someone with whom I could share my life.

It is a cold December morning in 1967; fresh snow lies everywhere. As I walk toward the car, the snow squeaks under my feet. My work at the hospital is far from my mind as I drive downtown to the Windsor Hotel. On Dominion Square, the white snow, the bright blue sky, the stark bare branches frame the stately building where I am to embark on a new adventure. I have been working at least fourteen hours a day during the past week as an intern in surgery, and I am exhausted—but this morning, a new world is opening up. It is my wedding day. Rhona and I have been going out for about a year. For the first time, a woman has been able to break through my fear of closeness, and I succumb to a peaceful tenderness that I had forgotten could exist.

My in-laws had reserved a suite in the hotel where we could change and take photographs prior to the ceremony and luncheon. The rooms were filled with people—my parents, Rhona's parents, my best man, the maid of honor, and finally, Rhona. When she entered the room in her wedding dress, her smile and warmth filled me with joy and fear. This was to be a bittersweet day.

My father began to pace shortly after the photographers began to pose us. I could see my mother admonish him and attempt to divert him from his ever-increasing anxiety. I looked around the room and hoped that no one else could see what was happening. He seemed distracted, and then, as the tension grew, he began to blow his nose—not once but many times. I tried to concentrate on my future wife, to feel only happiness, but the old rage at him, at the doctors, at life, knotted up my insides. I observed, as always, my mother's sadness and anxiety; the three of us once again played out a well-rehearsed and tragic scene. This time, however, there was a new role, an ingenue who stole the scene and saved my happiness. Rhona saw what was taking place; she took my hand and held it tightly, and my rage subsided. We went through the ceremony with joy. I tried not to look at my father, whose handkerchief was busy at his nose throughout. As we ran up the aisle, man and wife, I knew that I must let him go.

Yes, he had improved, but even on my wedding day, the past loomed like a specter over us as his residual difficulties came uninvited to the celebration.

5

Becoming a Psychiatrist

In September 1963, I entered medical school at McGill University. Imbued with high ideals, I hoped to become a healer filled with the kind of compassion that I thought characterized the lives of Norman Bethune—the McGill physician who contributed so much to the lives of both the Chinese and Spanish people—and Albert Schweitzer. On the outside, I looked like any other medical student, but the motivations that were driving me went far beyond the ideals I espoused. My life had been bound up with physicians and hospitals for eight years; I had spent many hours in the role of caretaker for my father. It was a role that I knew well. Being a physician allowed me the opportunity to continue to nurture and provide comfort for others; it also provided the possibility that I could, perhaps, heal disease—a possibility that had eluded the physicians who took care of my father. And so in my unconscious lay the wish to rework the past.

Medical school was a joyful experience. I began to gain confidence as a person; I could test my abilities and see my growth; I learned and I excelled. Although one of my reasons for entering medical school was to please my parents, I found that the fit was right, and I could pursue ideals that seemed worthwhile. I have no recollection of any exposure to psychiatry during the first two years of medical school. Interestingly, at my recent twentieth-year medical school reunion, several of my classmates reminded me that Ewen Cameron had lectured to us during our first year. I was shocked. How could it be that I had totally forgotten that I had seen or met the man whose experiments so changed the course of my life?

During my third year, I spent six weeks on a ward at the Allan Memorial Institute as a psychiatric clerk. This meant that I was assigned to two patients as a kind of junior doctor. I attended rounds, spoke with a supervisor, and went to lectures about current concepts of psychiatric care. Of all my clinical experiences in medical school, I remember least about this one. I do recollect that I was vigilant—I kept trying to discover clues about what had happened to my father—but I never went to see a shock treatment given, I did not ask about Ewen Cameron, and, as I have noted, I was not brave enough to examine my father's medical record. I continued to do more work in psychiatry during my senior year, but this time at a different hospital. Curiously enough, I did rather well and, on graduation, received a prize for great achievement in psychiatry. I was elated and felt that I had deserved the recognition, but although drawn to the field, I resisted and chose to consider other specialties as more suitable to my career goals. By this time I had so impressed people that I could have stayed at McGill to do a residency in pediatrics, surgery, or medicine. I was very torn, and I agonized over what was right for me. The uncertainty continued throughout my internship at the Montreal General Hospital.

Yet when I think about it now, there was really no choice to be made. Powerful forces were at work compelling me in the direction of psychiatry. My life had been taken up by the field for a long time; I had a burning need to understand what had taken place. In addition, I was filled with great fear about what psychiatrists could do. If I became one of them, I would no longer have to be afraid; I, too, would possess the secrets of power that could change people's lives.

There was likely the wish, as well, that if I had the knowledge, I might be able to undo the events of the previous ten years. I was aware that I could not pursue this track at McGill; it was a place filled with wretched memories. As the time approached to make a decision, I realized two things—I had to leave Montreal, and I had to become a psychiatrist.

It had taken a long time for me to be able to leave Montreal. I had long wanted to go away for university, but my parents merely pointed out the lack of funds. When the time came for medical school, I had not been accepted at any of the American schools to which I applied; I could not explain the precipitous drop in grades during my second year when we were forced to sell the house in which I had grown up. There was another problem, too. I had worked in Nova Scotia for three years during the summers, but whenever I did so I felt tremendously guilty for leaving my mother alone to cope with the difficulties of caring for my father. When I entered medical school, I moved out of our apartment and into a university residence. As a medical student, I had my own room in a building that had been completed only two years before. For the first time, I could walk to class no longer bothered by ice and snow or the other hassles of a commuting student. It should have been perfect. Here I was in medical school at last—new friends to meet, away from home, growing up. Yet when I tried to fall asleep on the first night, I was plagued by images of my parents—especially my mother, living with few friends and a husband who was barely a partner. I could not tolerate my feeling that I had abandoned her. Within six weeks I was home.

Two factors eventually allowed me to leave home again. First, I began to spend nights sleeping in the hospital as I worked on the wards. Second, by my fourth year I had met Rhona and my emotions turned elsewhere. I knew that I had to leave Montreal if I were to be free, and Yale provided the opportunity to do so.

I arrived in New Haven in July 1968 to begin a three-year residency in psychiatry at Yale University School of Medicine—seven years after my father's last hospitalization. Newly married, I was anticipating the opportunity to widen my world. The years in Connecticut were idyllic. Rhona was in graduate school while I trained as a psychiatrist. We lived in a red clapboard house about a hundred feet from the beach and Long Island Sound. I cannot imagine an environment more peaceful than our little beach house, far removed from Montreal with its pall of soul-destroying memories.

It might be reasonable to assume that, once in psychiatry, I would have attempted to learn more about what had happened to my father. I had the resources of a major library as well as faculty members who were among the most knowledgeable in the field. And yet I seemed to have put on blinders; I did not want to know. Once, I looked up a paper by Ewen Cameron, but so great was my need not to learn what my father had experienced that I cannot even remember which one it was.

Every so often I would be forced to confront the past. At least once a year my parents would drive down to visit. I looked forward to their arrival, each time hoping that it would be different, that my mother would be happy, my father well.

Each time I was disappointed. One year Rhona left school early to prepare a special meal for my parents—Rock Cornish hens with a Cumberland sauce. As we sat down, my father asked what the dish was. My mother tried to shush him up with a "Lou, whatever it is, you will enjoy it." He started to eat, then rose from the table and went to the bathroom. A few minutes later he returned. The ritual was repeated twice more. He picked up his fork and began to hum—a tuneless melody that accompanied his eating at every meal. Suddenly he began to spit the food into his napkin. "Feh," he exclaimed, "I can't eat this sauce. It's poison. How can you expect anyone to eat this stuff?"

I looked at my mother, at my wife, and at a man that I used to love. I was enraged. I wanted to run as I had when he was in the hospital—but there was no place to go. This was my home; I was no longer a child. Gone were the dinners at Ruby Foos; gone was the joyful embarrassment as he made us laugh. This is not my father, I prayed. But he was, and I watched helplessly as he continued to spit into the napkin. At that moment, the telephone rang and I gratefully rose to answer. When I returned a few minutes later, Rhona, in tears, sat with my mother finishing the meal. My father was outside on the screen porch smoking a cigar, pacing back and forth. I sat down and looked at them. I wanted to reach out and hold these two women that I loved, but I was frozen. Instead, we went on as always. What else could we do? Living with my father meant accepting what he had become—a petulant child in the body of a man.

The room had very little furniture—a desk against the wall, two chairs, a low coffee table, and a small bookcase. Gray walls, white tile floor, and a tall window completed the utilitarian, bland, and institutional decor. I had tried to enliven the room's appearance with photographs of the sea and with a black-and-white still of a young woman, her long hair caught by a breeze and her face in a shadow. That photograph burns in my memory as I picture my first office as a psychiatry resident. The young woman reminds me of so many of the troubled adolescents that I worked with during the late 1960s. Young people who were running away, taking all the fashionable drugs of the time, hiding from their parents, their teachers, and most of all, themselves. LSD, mushrooms, mescaline, uppers, downers, "luudes," marijuana, MDA, STP—the initials tripped off the lips of these flower children as they sunk deeper into the depths of confusion and, often, despair.

I felt a special attachment to them because their pain evoked an echo in me. I responded to them with my own feelings of loss, with memories of walking along fog-shrouded streets at night, seeing families together in lighted windows and wishing that I, too, could belong. I was a casualty as well, but I could use my pain to help them.

The heat was almost unbearable, despite the air-conditioning. I felt my eyes closing and I fought to stay awake as the patient droned on. My thoughts kept moving away from his words; I could not concentrate, no matter how hard I tried. It was the second month of residency and I was trying to learn how to sit still and listen to my patients. After a year of constant work and pressure as an intern, I was finding it very difficult to adapt to the slower pace of psychiatry.

What's the matter with me? Why am I so tired? I wish that I were back in the O.R. What is he saying? It is so hot. I can't seem to listen to him.

"Doctor, I don't sleep. I feel so bad all the time. My legs hurt, and my back. Can't you do anything for me? I might as well kill myself; no one would care anyway." He rose and began to pace the room, wringing his hands. His whining voice persisted in its complaints: "I've always been a good man. I worked hard all my life. Maybe I made some mistakes; maybe I wasn't always as honest as I should have been. Why is God punishing me? Doctor, can't you give me some medicine?" His crying was loud and accompanied by sobs that seemed to shake his entire body.

I should feel sorry for him—but I feel distant. It's just that I'm so tired. All right, what's wrong with him? He hasn't been sleeping for a month; he wakes up at 4:00 A.M. every day and lies in bed thinking that his life has been a waste. He hasn't been able to eat, and has lost about thirteen pounds. Although he says that he has no energy, his wife told me that he is constantly wandering around the house crying and moaning. They have not had sexual relations for more than a month; he says that he is too sick. All right, he's depressed. He thinks that his partner wants him out—is he a little paranoid? What kind of depression is this—psychotic or not? If I were to use medications, what would I use? Why do I feel so angry around this guy?

Joseph Minotti was a fifty-four-year-old first-generation Italian-American man, born into a blue-collar family in New Haven. New York was the farthest he had been since he was born. He had struggled to build a small business that had in fact succeeded beyond his dreams during the previous three years, and for a while, he, his wife Carla, and their four daughters had led a very comfortable existence. Joseph was short, balding, and very fat. He no longer cared about his appearance and his disheveled attire, coupled with his runny nose and weepy eyes, made him a sorry sight. His irritability and helplessness played havoc with my feelings about him as a patient—one minute, I empathized with him, the next, I wanted him out of my office. I couldn't understand why this sad little man was affecting me in such an unusual manner. I began to blame myself for not caring enough; I would avoid him in the hallway; my sessions with him felt never ending, and as his irritability rose, I would withdraw and sleepiness would beckon.

The time-honored approach to learning psychotherapy is to present your therapy hours to a senior psychiatrist who acts as your supervisor. After each session, I would dutifully try to remember what had happened during the hour, and write it all down on paper. "I said . . . and Mr. Minotti said . . . and I felt . . . and Mr. Minotti began to cry. . . ." For a long time, I never told my supervisor that I couldn't keep my eyes open during the therapy, or that I felt very angry at this patient.

One day, Mr. Minotti accused me of being a useless doctor, of being totally unable to help him get better. I felt very agitated; I reviewed his medications and my work with him and his wife. I was doing all the right things—why did I feel so bad? As I talked to my supervisor, I felt a rush of emotion and tears wet my cheeks—it wasn't Mr. Minotti whom I could not help, it was my father. Each time that I walked into the office with my patient, it was my father who sat down across from me. I became sleepy to avoid listening to him. The self-doubts arose out of memories of my helplessness. The anger came from two sources: first, I was angry at myself for being a bad doctor ("son"); second, I was angry at him for being a bad patient ("father") who would not get well. I could not reveal all of this to the supervisor, but by talking about my difficulties in listening, the truth became apparent. Afterward, it was as though my head had just cleared. I could talk with Joseph, I could feel for him, and he improved.

With Rhona as support, I was now able to involve myself with people in a way that I had never previously allowed. The freedom to make friends resulted in the development of relationships that, fifteen years later, still constitute a major source of pleasure in my life. Even so, I began to realize that I was ambivalent about my chosen specialty. Given the underlying motivation to become part of a field that had brought me so much pain, it is apparent that I could not do so without accepting its role in the destruction of my father's life. To accept that was untenable. I thought about leaving psychiatry and returning to internal medicine or pediatrics. I persisted, but every so often the past emerged and I was confronted with the darkness inside.

I awoke with a headache. The room was still dark; I could not remember the dream that had frightened me. My heart was racing and there was sweat on my forehead. I reached over to hold my wife, but I could not calm myself. The scream was still lodged in my throat, ready to explode in rage. Yet, I was silent. As I began to relax, the realization began to crystallize. Today was the day that I would learn to give shock treatment, electroconvulsive therapy, ECT. What was I going to do? I had never shied away from anything that I feared; in fact, one characteristic of my personality had been that I always challenged myself with what I feared the most. But shock treatment: I sat up and tried to make a decision. Could I go through with it? Yesterday, the chief resident had come into my office and told me that ECT was the only reasonable choice left for Greta, my patient. Medications had not worked; psychotherapy was not the answer. Fragments of my dream returned, and as they did, I suddenly became very afraid. The last image before I awoke was of my hand reaching out. I looked at the clock beside the bed—still two hours before I had to get up. My chief had scheduled the ECT for the morning.

ECT had previously been discussed with Greta, but I usually reassured her that antidepressant medications would do the trick. I suppose that I had not wanted to admit that I, as a psychiatrist, might have to push the button that discharged electricity into the brain of my patient. Intellectually, I knew the efficacy of the treatment; the literature was complete and definitive. Controversy about the possibility of brain damage still existed, but, in the limited amounts that were now used, the only organic problem would be a transient memory loss.

The evening before, at my chief's suggestion, I had visited Greta to tell her of our decision that ECT was needed, and to have her sign the consent form. She was alone, staring out the window at the darkening sky. I told her of the decision and she shrugged her shoulders, "You're the doctors." I tried once again to explain why ECT was needed and the possible side effects. Once more she said, "Fine, do what you have to." She signed the consent form and as I left the room I realized that this was much more difficult for me than for her. That night I reread my material on shock and thought about a man confused, incontinent, and helpless.

I arrived at my office early and went in to say hello to the patient. She had already received some premedication and was quiet. The chief resident came in and asked if I was ready; I smiled and said that I was, while inside, I thought that I would never be able to go through with it. He showed me the machine—small, seemingly innocuous—and pointed to the button. It is strange sometimes how a fragment of your vision—a flower, a color, a piece of jewelry, something that has a great deal of meaning for you—seems to grow and fill up your sight, as though the rest of the world is of no significance at all. And so, for a while, the button became the focus of my life: I pressed it, and then the treatment was over.

That was the only time that I gave a shock treatment. It was not so terrible an experience; in fact, Greta did quite well and after a few treatments made a rapid recovery. I knew, however, that I could never press that button again. I asked a colleague to do the treatments for me without explaining the reasons; I told the chief resident that I would not give ECT, and he accepted that. What did I feel afterward? Relief, sadness, and likely resignation because the past was the past, and I could not change the course of my father's life. His time had come and gone.

The first months of my residency were a disaster, as I attempted to assimilate and deal with the process of residency training. The focus on psychological motivation, rather than being a welcome concept, became a piece of gristle, undigestible food that would stick in my throat. In addition, my security as a physician was shattered. Symptom relief was often so slow, cure frequently impossible. I felt that I was inwardly rebelling against the changes that were being demanded of me as my ticket into the profession.

One of the reasons that psychiatry had seemed like a good fit for me was that I had seen it as a career pathway that would not only allow me to express my professional expertise, but also encourage me to think and feel. By the middle of my medical internship year, I had begun to feel distanced from patients. Always tired, I still felt a real sense of exhilaration because I was effective—people improved, symptoms disappeared. At the same time, however, what I lost in medical school and internship was the opportunity for involvement; in the rush of reading and doing, I had lost the sense of being. Psychiatry, I thought, would restore it. I had not bargained on the changes that I would have to undergo as I shifted from a focus on the body to one on the mind.

Throughout most of this century, specializing in psychiatry has required that the trainee move from the model of diseased organs to that of a possibly diseased mind—a much more abstruse entity. Consequently, psychiatric residents in their first year were forced to confront their identities as physicians as they found themselves both respected for medical expertise and denigrated for lack of psychological expertise. For me, it became increasingly difficult to maintain the concept of myself as a physician, and I fought the changes that becoming a psychiatrist required. I was torn. During that year I also began to realize just how much my father was going to be part of my career. By choosing psychiatry, I again had chosen to confront that which I feared. The repercussions of that choice were to stay with me.

I had other problems too. In 1968, when I began my residency, psychiatry was still caught up in the turbulent social changes that characterized the late 1960s. Wherever I had gone to interview for residency programs, a race riot had occurred within the previous year. Minority communities were demanding better and more relevant services from psychiatrists; the community mental health movement was at its zenith; paraprofessionals from the community were invited to become therapists and move upward on a ladder to nowhere, since job opportunities were limited. When I entered this chaos, I was totally lost. For the first time, I began to realize how different a country the United States was from my own. Trying to reconcile all the usual issues of becoming a psychiatrist with the social issues of civil rights was a formidable task.

When my mixed feelings about psychiatry continued to grow, I decided to resign from the residency and contacted the training director. He confirmed for me what until then I had only suspected—that my anxiety arose from the chaos within the institution, and not from any disturbance within myself. What was apparent, however, was that my acute sensitivity to the troubled relationships within the training setting grew out of the intense experience over the years of observing my father and the family.

After long discussion, I chose to continue, but for the first time sought psychotherapy to try to sort out my concerns about becoming a psychiatrist.

When I entered the therapist's office for the first time, I was faced with a significant dilemma. Should I open the Pandora's box of horrors that surged and battered my insides? Or should I focus instead on the immediate question of career? I quickly became aware that I lived with the constant fear that I would "go crazy." At that time, I had no other explanation for what had destroyed my father, and I lived with the nightmare that the darkness would be mine as well.

In psychotherapy, I went over the events of my adolescence, and my fear gradually receded as I saw how different I was from my father. As weeks passed, I told the story in many different ways, each time recalling images that I had thought were banished from awareness. The warm encouragement of my therapist facilitated my remembering; his ready acceptance of my rage and hurt provided the opportunity to move on. Life, for me, had stopped when I was fourteen, but I was now twenty-six years old. With each telling, the pain receded. As I explored the memories of my father and those dark days in the 1950s, I began to see the impossible position into which I had placed myself. Becoming a psychiatrist meant becoming a colleague of Ewen Cameron. The sources of my ambivalence became very clear. Over the next two years, the healing benefits of the therapeutic process allowed me to confront the nameless fears, and I thought that I would be able to devote myself to the field I had chosen.

During this period I did quite well as a resident. I was offered a prestigious Chief Residency (which I turned down in order to work intensively with disturbed adolescents) and was highly spoken of by my supervisors. Yet I began to notice a pattern that was as disturbing as it was consistent. I would gain the respect of those in authority, and then either back away or else attack them on an issue that had merit but which I could only lose, fighting from a position of powerlessness. This pattern was to haunt me for a very long time. I gradually began to understand that its origins lay in my relationship to a father who was lost, and to a profession that had stolen him from me without explanation. My decision to enter psychiatry, I now realized, arose from a need to understand what had taken place and, further, to gain control over my anger toward psychiatry by becoming part of the profession myself. Unfortunately, I could not control the rage that would periodically erupt. My father's ordeal at the Allan Memorial had to become a significant part of my adult life experience; his pain had been transmitted to the next generation.

As we finished our education and training at Yale, a decision had to be made about where we would live. Rhona preferred the East where she could be near her parents; I felt as though the four hundred miles between Montreal and New Haven were not far enough. Three thousand miles seemed about right at that point, and San Francisco became our new home. I still remember the morning that we set out from Montreal for the drive west. Both sets of parents stood waving in the driveway; my mother and mother-in-law were in tears; Rhona sobbed beside me. I felt a gut-wrenching pull as I drove down the familiar streets. This time it felt final; my only thought was escape. I left a great part of myself behind.

We settled into our new lives—Rhona became a professor at the University of California in Berkeley and I practiced as a psychiatrist in San Francisco. Three years later, an event occurred which had a major impact on me. In 1975, Rhona gave birth to our twin sons. We had been married for eight years and the timing seemed right. I threw myself into the preparations, and when my sons were born I arranged my schedule so that I only needed to miss one feeding a day. I found that I could not stand to be away from them. Our friends and colleagues marveled at the extent of my involvement, and we became to many the paragon of the true two-career couple. And yet, I began to realize that once again there were forces at work over which I had no control. Up to this time, I had been traveling often for work—presenting papers, working on grants, and the like—now I was afraid to travel. Suffering recurrent nightmares that the airplane would crash and my children would grow up without a father, I found myself avoiding meetings that were out of town. I again began to worry that I, too, would succumb to whatever the illness was that took my father away from me. I felt that I had to give as much to my children as possible before I turned fifty because by then I might be a lethargic shell, totally self-absorbed and unable to respond to the needs of my family.

At the same time, conflicts arose in my professional life. In the mid-1970s, I was director of a psychiatry residency training program, the focus of which was to develop an educational methodology where clear expectations and objective evaluation would both enhance learning and help to alleviate the anxiety engendered by the process of becoming a psychiatrist. The program was very exciting; grants were obtained and national recognition was at hand. To my dismay, however, the old pattern emerged; problems between my mentor and myself led to my seeking psychotherapy from a man who finally helped me to let go of the past.

His office was on the second floor of a stone mansion on one of San Francisco's most lovely streets. His wife, also a psychiatrist, had an office one floor above, and they lived in the upper stories with windows that opened out to the Bay and the hills of Marin County. As I mounted the steps through the fiery red bougainvillea and the lush foliage that cascaded down the hillside and through the arches, I felt a great sense of defeat.

You'll never be happy. Your life will never be what you wanted it to. You are destined to go through your days peering through windows; eavesdropping on the lives of those who live their dreams. . . .

I rang the bell and was admitted to a waiting room. Everything was still. On the walls were hangings from Latin America; on the table, copies of the latest news magazines and some quality periodicals. I couldn't get much of a sense of him from my surroundings. I was very anxious and filled with anticipation as I waited.

I heard the sound of steps and the front door closed abruptly, leaving me with the roar of silence. More steps, and a silver-haired man, tall and stately, thin, almost cadaverous in appearance, entered the room. After the appropriate introductions, we went up to his office and he motioned me to sit down. It was a peaceful place—walls of books, oriental rugs, a couch across from me and two chairs. The window revealed the beauty of the Bay and the Golden Gate Bridge. The fog was just beginning to be sucked into the Gate, and I could glimpse wisps of white against the blue of the sky and the stark gold of the Marin hills. I fixed my eye on a slim volume of poetry by Rainer Maria Rilke and, for the first time, I told my story, with the understanding that my career as a psychiatrist depended on coming to terms with what had happened to my father.

As months passed, the message became an imperative; "You are responsible for your own life." For years I felt guilty about the feelings I had toward my father. I held on to the guilt like a shield—using it to justify my passivity in the face of adversity. I saw the world as an unfair place, but rather than fight I would give up responsibility because I saw myself as helpless. "I am not responsible for what happened to him. . . ." Yes, I encouraged my mother to send him back, but I was only a kid. . . . Yes, there were times that I hated him and never wanted to see him again, but that was a normal response. . . . I don't have the sole obligation to make up to them all that has happened; I have a wife and two new children . . . but it hurts. God, how it hurts.

Over the next two years, I railed against this gentle man. I wept; I thundered; I felt the need to be close; I saw my fear of the closeness. Within the confines of that lovely room, the world of my adolescence became alive once more as I struggled to become a man. Never did he let me feel sorry for myself. "You must live in the present. How are you going to deal with the politics at work?" "If you feel isolated, what are you going to do about it?" His patience and gentle manner enabled me to let go of my preoccupation with the past. My anger at psychiatry could focus on one institution and one man. From my therapist I gained the freedom to follow my profession; unencumbered, I could use my life experience in ways that would assist others.

Looking back now on my youth through the long telescope of experience, I understand that my father's sense of helplessness and anger had been transmitted to me; the dark cloud over his head had become my own. I also realize that, because I had felt the obligation to assuage the hurt, my career choice was determined. This ultimately led to profound internal struggle as I sought to involve myself with psychiatry on terms with which I felt comfortable. How many of us find ourselves in careers because we are living out another's dream or nightmare?

In the mid-1970s, despite the insights and relief I had gained through therapy, I was burdened with a sense of failure—too many questions remained unanswered. My father had changed beyond recognition and our lives had been altered beyond imagining, but with all of my psychiatric knowledge I was still in ignorance as to why it had happened. The best explanation I could come up with was that my father's suffering was a bad response to standard treatment—an unfortunate outcome of routine procedures.

Three years later, in 1979, I had the first hint that a different explanation was possible. The enormity of what had transpired, the awful truth of research funded by the governments of the United States and Canada, the abuse of patients in the name of science—it all exploded before my eyes in a small item in a newspaper, and the search for justice began.

Part 2: Discovery

6

My Awakening

There is an old Yiddish expression that my grandmother used to say. It translates roughly as follows: "You should only grow like an onion—with your head in the ground." When I first read *The Search for the Manchurian Candidate*, John Marks's exposé of the CIA mind-control experiments, I felt as though my head had been buried for a very long time. I had wasted years diagnosing my father with a variety of psychotic labels; I had blamed myself; I had perused the psychiatric literature in a lame search for answers that could not be found. I had read a couple of Cameron's articles, but their significance had not penetrated my thinking. Perhaps I never wanted to lift my head out of the mud; maybe I was afraid that the truth would prove to be even more painful than the memories.

In the spring of 1979, shortly after my discovery of CIA funding of Ewen Cameron's work, I wrote John Marks a letter asking how I could learn more about this subject, and more specifically, about my father's involvement in the program. In his reply, he expressed his sadness over what had happened to my father and also raised an issue that I had never considered: "I think that you are much more likely to get some satisfaction by a direct suit against the government. Indeed, I know two lawyers who have expressed interest in representing clients in such a suit, and I have referred two other patients of Cameron to one of them. I am taking the liberty of sending your letter on to the lawyers. . . ."

The thought of a lawsuit was totally foreign to me. It was also clear that my father felt so much shame and guilt about the experience that a lawsuit would potentially be quite debilitating. Still, I had recently learned that my mother had sold some pieces of fine china so that they could have extra cash, and that the sterling silver was going to be next. While I felt that no amount of money could compensate for wasted years, I began to think how wonderful it would be if the last years of my parents' lives could be free of monetary pressures. Even more important to me, however, was the hope that my father would be vindicated—that he could lose the sense of shame. No longer would he have to feel that he was guilty of some wrongdoing. As for me, I am not, by nature, a litigious person; the thought of lawyers and courtrooms made me very hesitant to consider a lawsuit.

I fretted and procrastinated about this, and kept it, as usual, to myself. In the late spring of 1980, I mentioned to my mother that I had read a book that revealed a link between Ewen Cameron and the CIA. When she mentioned it to my father, he responded at first with a shrug of disbelief, and then became increasingly agitated. Clearly, no discussion was possible. I doubted that he even understood what the issues were. My mother was very distressed, both about the revelations and about my father's inability to deal with this news. After a particularly upsetting conversation with her, I decided that there was no point in pursuing the matter. At that point, any further discussion was cut short by the sudden death of my brother-in-law, Dan. Our lives were quickly taken up by my sister's needs, and I never really had the opportunity to discuss the revelations of CIA involvement with my father.

In August 1980, I received a letter from the man who was to occupy a considerable part of my thoughts and emotions for the next few years. The letter read:

> We represent a group of Canadian citizens who are considering suit against the U.S. Central Intelligence Agency because of "treatment" they received while under the care of Dr. D. Ewen Cameron at the Allan Memorial Institute. About two years ago, the CIA revealed that it had funded Dr. Cameron's research at the Allan Institute under project MKULTRA, a top secret program that supplied money to researchers investigating various techniques of behavior control and brainwashing.

The letter went on to request my assistance by providing information about what had transpired at McGill. It was signed by a man named Joseph L. Rauh, Jr., a Washington attorney.

So it really is going to happen, I thought; some people have the guts to fight. I subsequently found out that the drive for justice was spearheaded by a man named David Orlikow, a member of the Canadian Parliament (similar to a United States congressman), whose wife, Val, had been a patient of Cameron's for several years. Mr. Orlikow, following the revelations of American government funding at the Allan Memorial, had sought an American attorney to help institute a suit. The Orlikow's had previously brought suit against the Allan Memorial Institute and the Royal Victoria Hospital in Montreal, a case that was ultimately settled out of court. The attorney that was suggested to the Orlikow's was Joe Rauh.

Mr. Rauh had a reputation as one of the foremost civil rights attorneys in the United States. Harvard-trained, he had served as a law clerk for two of the most distinguished jurists of the American legal system, Benjamin Cardozo and Felix Frankfurter. He had devoted his career and considerable talents to championing the civil liberties of American citizens. He had served as counsel to the United Auto Workers, the Miners for Democracy, the Leadership Conference for Civil Rights, and had represented Arthur Miller and Lillian Hellman before the infamous House Un-American Activities Committee, whose work extended the destructive "red-baiting" of Senator Joseph McCarthy. With the assistance of the Center for National Security Studies (an affiliate of the American Civil Liberties Union) and some publicity, attempts were made to alert other patients of Ewen Cameron. Those who came forward were invited to participate in a multiple-plaintiff suit against the CIA.

During the next year, my mother tried to talk with my father about the importance of fighting this case in court. She got nowhere. The effects of the "treatment" that my father received at the Allan Memorial made it difficult for him to cope with this issue. Basically, his condition is marked by a peculiar rigidity of thinking. Thus, he will make up his mind very quickly, and further discussion is impossible. This is likely a legacy of massive electroconvulsive shock treatment, drugs, forced sleep, sensory deprivation, and anoxia (lack of oxygen). Combined with this symptom is extreme passivity, a lack of will that probably grew out of the profound sense of helplessness he had felt for many years. In many situations, he simply cannot make a decision and is paralyzed until pushed in one direction or another. To further compound the difficulty, he is quite capable of feelings, and he lives with a constant sense that he is a failure. The shame that this evoked, on top of the chronic problems that the years at the Allan Memorial had bestowed, made it impossible for him to consider participation in a lawsuit.

In these circumstances, I had to accept my own helplessness in the situation. Periodically, I would raise the issue, but finally my mother told me to stop. Whenever we would end our telephone conversations in which I had pursued the topic, my father would become very anxious and depressed. He would become silent and morose and take to the couch with his cigar; the tension would last for days. At her request, I gave up.

On October 17, 1981, the telephone rang as I was leaving to take my son to an art lesson. It was a sunny Saturday morning, but on that day some of the sunshine disappeared from my life. My brother-in-law, Leon, told me that earlier in the morning my mother had awakened with chest pain. She did not tell my father for a long time until at breakfast he noticed that she was very quiet and not eating. When she told him, they tried to reach their physician but having no success, decided to go to the local hospital emergency room. It was so characteristic of my mother that before they left she made both my father's bed and her own, and cleared and washed the breakfast dishes. Even as the end approached, she did not relinquish her role as his caretaker. I am convinced that she knew what was happening.

Events then occurred very quickly. My father drove to the hospital at breakneck speed, not stopping at traffic lights; they talked very little. On arrival, she was whisked away behind closed doors. An intern told my father that she was experiencing a heart attack. He telephoned my sisters and brother-in-law, and they rushed to the emergency room to be with him.

It was over within two hours. My parents never said goodbye.

I flew to Montreal in a daze. For years, I had cherished the fantasy that, since my father was older than my mother, she would outlive him; on his death, she would then have the opportunity to devote some time to herself. In my head, I used to plan her visits to California and anticipate the pleasure that she and all of us would have. As the plane flew east, I was filled with an ache; my dream had once again become a nightmare. The future became the present and the present was filled with a longing that would never be satisfied.

At the funeral, I spoke about her: "My mother was solid and loyal. She stood by my father in the bad times. She gave him strength; he gave her adoration. Firmly grounded, she never wavered. Through my adolescence, she propped us up and never complained. As a life companion, she gave her husband the sustenance he needed to rebuild his life. She was wife—giver of strength."

During the obligatory seven days of mourning that is part of Jewish ritual, I stayed with my father in the apartment. The house was always full of people bringing food, memories, and warmth. I kept expecting my mother to appear suddenly out of the kitchen, or to answer the front door to let me in. Beside her bed was a book she would never finish; her knitting rested in a bag beside her chair.

On the eighth day, at six in the morning, I arose in darkness. My flight to California was at eight o'clock; I had to return to work. My father came out of his room in his bathrobe and watched as I closed up the hide-a-bed and made coffee. We talked about my life in California, and how he would spend the day. We talked of people, and food. We talked of my sisters and my children. We never talked about loss.

At 7:15, I knew that I had to go downstairs for the taxi, and we embraced. He was a tough old bird then. Faced with overwhelming loneliness, he showed no pain as I entered the elevator and waved goodbye. I could barely contain the sadness inside; it felt as though I was abandoning him. California, here I come, I thought.

My father wandered through the next months alone and dazed. I began to feel that he should not live out the rest of his years without righting the terrible wrong that was done to him at the Allan Memorial Institute. I felt that if he could fight for something and be made to understand that the limitations on his life were a result of the injuries that he had suffered at the Institute, it would help him in the days ahead. Toward the end of 1981, I began again to talk with my father about fighting the case in Washington. At first tentatively, then more insistently, I tried to help him understand what the case meant, both for him and in its broader context. Finally, he contacted Mr. Rauh, and I learned to my horror that there was a question as to whether he could participate in the suit. Because he had heard of the CIA involvement in 1980 but had only instituted a claim in 1982, his case might have exceeded the statute of limitations. I wrote to Mr. Rauh:

> It somehow seems very ironic to me that my father, who through the "treatment" rendered by the CIA is rendered unable to follow through with a lawsuit because of paralysis of will, is then prevented from carrying out a suit by the statute of limitations. Even though my father had the information, the treatment had so incapacitated him that he was unable to act until only recently. . . . If one purpose of the lawsuit is to focus attention on unethical medical practice funded by a United States government agency whereby the minds of individuals were manipulated and profoundly changed, then how can one expect such a victim to be able to process the

knowledge of wrongdoing and act accordingly, in the same way as a psychologically healthy person?

My argument appeared to carry some weight because the lawyers agreed to review the files from the Allan Memorial (some five hundred pages) and consider taking on my father as a client.

By December 1982, my father had become a participant in a multiple-plaintiff suit against the Central Intelligence Agency of the United States. The suit—*Orlikow vs. the United States of America*—was filed in the United States District Court for the District of Columbia. Six Canadians were part of the original complaint; three more (including my father) were to follow. The *Toronto Star* (August 18, 1985) profiled the plaintiffs as follows:

1. Velma Orlikow: wife of Winnipeg member of Parliament David Orlikow. "Under Cameron's supervision, her suit alleges she was given LSD 14 times during 1956 and 1957 and was forced to undergo 'psychic driving.' . . . At first she was subjected to the tapes for periods of four hours at a time, but until she refused to continue as an outpatient in December 1963, she had been undergoing psychic driving six hours each day. She has suffered sporadic debilitating depression since."
2. Jean-Charles Page: "Under Cameron's supervision, Page was given a variety of drugs and given 30 straight days days of psychic driving plus 36 consecutive days of induced sleep."
3. Robert Logie: "He too was given LSD, a variety of other drugs, shock treatment and spent twenty-three days in induced sleep. 'I can't sleep at night—I haven't been able to sleep for more than three hours a night since they put me to sleep for those twenty-three days.' "
4. Jeanine Huard: "Given electroshock and psychic driving."
5. Lydia Stadler: "Had one of the longest stays at the Allan, from 1954 to treatment as an outpatient in 1964. Her

mental injuries are regarded as permanent and Stadler is now in an institution."

6. Mary Morrow: "Depatterned with massive electroconvulsive treatments."
7. Rita Zimmerman: "Given 56 days of 'sleep treatment' and 30 electroshock treatments between July 3 and September 22, 1959, to the point where she was so depatterned Cameron noted she had become 'incontinent of stool on occasion.' "
8. Florence Langleben: "Returned [to the Allan] August 20, 1959, and from that date until November 6, 1959, the suit alleges, she received a total of 43 days of drug-induced sleep, 15 electroconvulsive shock treatments, 32 days of negative psychic driving and 11 days of positive psychic driving."
9. Louis Weinstein: a man with "no life. He lost everything."

These nine Canadians, bound together by misfortune, were likely very similar to the more than one hundred that, by the count of Allan researchers, had participated in the depatterning/psychic-driving program. Where are the others? Some may be dead; others may be too incapacitated to come forward; a few may have no memory of the treatment. I expect that many were like my father—so ashamed of the experience that the thought of public exposure was a possibility that could not be contemplated.

Finally, I felt as though I had allies in righting an unspeakable injustice. Yet I still was unaware of what really had transpired at Allan Memorial. In 1983, I began to open my eyes; I started to read what I had half-pretended did not exist. For the first time, I began to review the published papers of Ewen Cameron. Through papers and references that I received from Rauh and his associate, Jim Turner, I embarked on a voyage of discovery. The words on paper were those that I had heard as an adolescent—sleep treatment, psychic driving, shock treatment—and more. I held myself in check, and only very slowly did I allow the beginnings of understanding to emerge. I found myself making notes—I wasn't at all sure what I was going to do with them, but I felt that I needed to record my ever-increasing knowledge.

In April 1985, Jim Turner called and asked me if I would

agree to appear on the CBS television program "Sixty Minutes." The old sense of helplessness swept over me, and I remember wondering whether anyone in the United States would care that lives of Canadians had been destroyed through CIA money and direction. This time, however, I felt ready to talk; I was prepared to express my anger and to act as a spokesman for many who could not talk, who might never come forward. I felt that, as a psychiatrist, I could explain what had been done; as a son, I could describe how callous disregard for humanity could rob a family of any reason for living.

In June, I went to the Clift Hotel in San Francisco. I sat in the lobby, sweating, anxious, reading and rereading the copious notes that I had made about Ewen Cameron and his work. Finally, I went up to the suite that CBS had reserved for the taping. Little did I know that this would be my initiation into the world of the media—the first of many interviews on radio, television, for magazines and newspapers. The door opened. There were lights, people milling about. I was welcomed by the woman who had been in touch with me, and then I felt superfluous. She and the producer went to the other room to discuss what they were going to shoot; the men setting up continued to move furniture around. "Sit here." I sat.

"Put the microphone on." I did.

"Talk."

About what? Why am I here? Is this happening? If I expected compassion or empathy, they were conspicuously absent. Finally, I was introduced to the interviewer. He was smooth, pleasant, chatty, and I felt at ease for a short while. We discussed some of his questions and I learned about how others saw the story. Sensational, an exposé—well, isn't that what "Sixty Minutes" does? When the lights went on and the tape began to roll, the interviewer metamorphosed into a "personality." Although his smooth style was off-putting, I persisted in trying to answer the questions. As time went on, however, I realized that much of what I had prepared would never be told. Two and a half hours; the tape whirred and stopped; on and off; speak and relax; remember and forget; remember, remember, never let it go.

The program was aired in December 1985, two days before

Christmas when the viewing audience was small. I appeared for two minutes refuting the statement by another psychiatrist that, because "these people were sick," their claims could be dismissed. We watched the program in a rented cottage on the ocean, one hundred and twenty miles from San Francisco. The sky was purple and orange with the setting winter sun; the Pacific was black, and so was my mood as I recalled all that had not been aired. A few minutes later, my oldest friend from Montreal called. Although he now lives in New York, he had traced us down and wanted to express his thoughts about the program. Little did I know that his was the first of many letters and calls from across North America.

Over the next months—calls from former patients and colleagues; letters from college students, the old and young; letters that were supportive, some that were psychotic and poisonous. I also began to hear from others that had been hurt by drug experiments—either directly, or indirectly because their father, brother, or friend had been involved—and I found myself swept up in their stories. I naively thought that all the information now coming to light would surely bring justice. All of these concerned people were an indication that American outrage would expedite the case to a successful conclusion. Of course, it died down. There are so many stories, so much tragedy—ho hum, another holocaust tale. How inured we are to debility, death, and degradation. The pain was mine alone; no one else could feel it; no one else could fight.

I gave talks. I spoke to more than a hundred Stanford students in a psychology class; I addressed many more in a public forum. I began to read voraciously about every aspect of what had transpired, my reading taking me to places that I had never thought relevant to my father's story. More television, more interviews—I was swept up in thinking about Ewen Cameron and I began to wonder who he was. What kind of man, what kind of physician would treat people in this manner? Questions began to percolate through my mind at all hours of the day and night—questions of ethics, of medical practice, of power and its abuses. I began to toy with the idea of writing a book, and the tempo increased.

As my communications with the lawyers increased, I found myself in libraries at every spare moment. Slowly I began to put the pieces of the puzzle together. Fragments from the psychiatric literature blended with the thoughts of those who had worked with Ewen Cameron; the deafening silence from those who would not talk with me contrasted markedly with those whose lives had been destroyed. By the winter of 1985, Ewen Cameron's work was less of an unknown; I had grown to know it well. But his person remained an enigma.

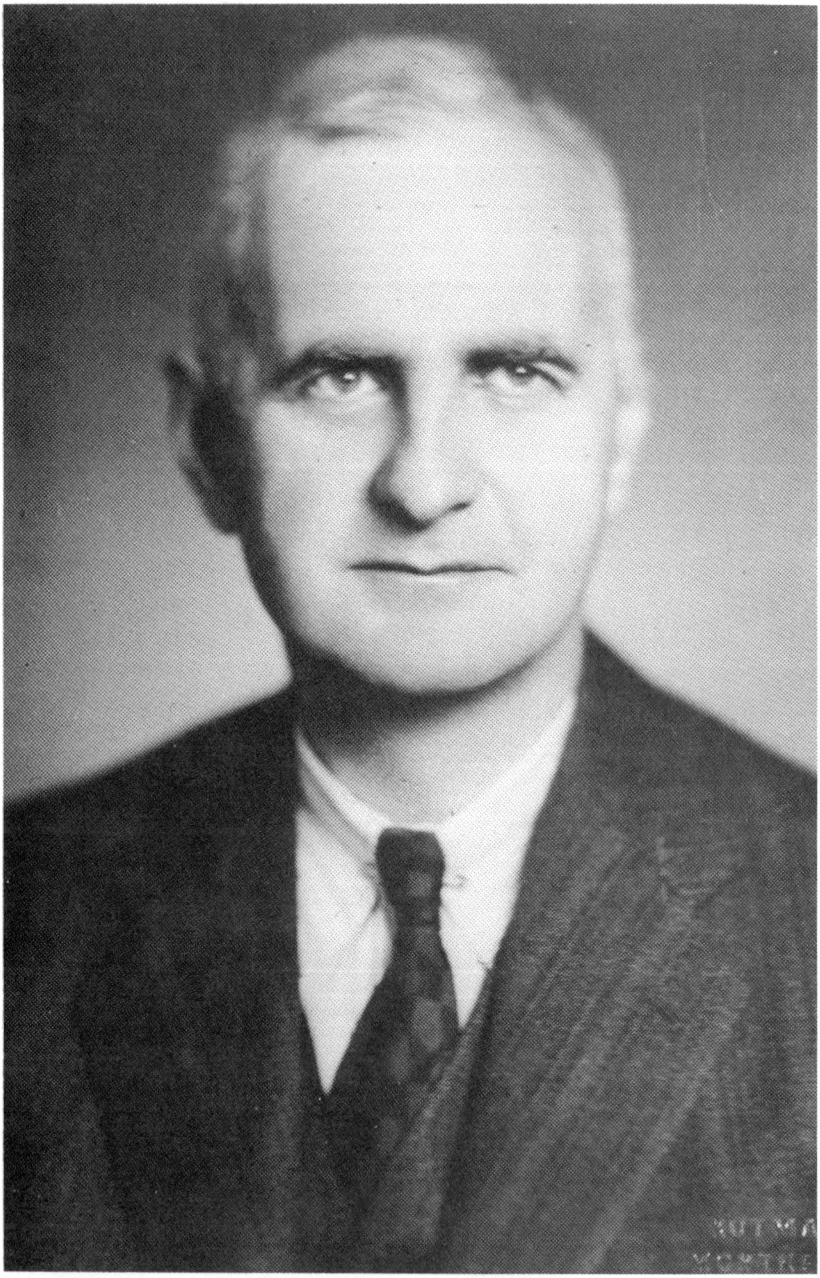

My father's doctor: Ewen Cameron, M.D., *c.* 1959–60 *(The American Psychiatric Association, Washington D.C.)*

7

My Father's Doctor: Ewen Cameron, M.D.

Who was this man, this shadowy figure who looms over the life of my father and haunts my life as well? During 1985, I found myself thinking about him more and more. It was as though, for thirty years, another man had joined our family, a man with greater influence and power than any of the rest of us. I was determined to discover and piece together a picture of the kind of physician who could become involved with the CIA and who would use his patients in experimentation. In order to understand a man who had been dead for almost twenty years, I would first have to talk with those who knew him; I would read all the papers that he had published in the professional journals; I would try to find his personal papers. The latter two tasks were easy enough—the Stanford Medical Library had all the journals that I required and the archives of the American Psychiatric Association held a collection of Cameron's papers. Unfortunately, many of his papers had been destroyed by his son and only those papers remaining had been deposited with the archives.

Finding psychiatrists or other mental health professionals to talk with me about the man proved a far more difficult task. Letters went unanswered; telephone calls were either avoided or secretaries informed me to call again, and again, and again. There were outright refusals to talk, especially from some of Cameron's coauthors. I realized that if I had tried to interview these people in 1977 at the time of the revelations, it would have been far easier. By 1986, lawsuits had been filed and the media in Canada were actively digging into the work of Ewen Cameron and the Allan Memorial Institute. I was told that the director of the Institute had instructed his staff not to talk. I did, however, find several people who were willing at least to attempt to address the issues that Cameron's work had raised. In addition, I had access to interviews that were carried out in 1977–78 by a researcher gathering data for John Marks's book. These filled in the picture.

Donald Ewen Cameron (he was commonly referred to as Ewen) was born in Bridge of Allan, Scotland, in 1901, the son of a Presbyterian minister. His Scottish education culminated in 1925 when he received his diploma in psychological medicine. That same year, at the Royal Mental Hospital in Glasgow, he became influenced by Sir David Henderson, who, in turn, had been taught by Adolph Meyer—a psychiatrist whose broadened perspective on psychiatry was to influence Cameron for the rest of his life. In 1926, Cameron left for America to work with Meyer at the Phipps Clinic at Johns Hopkins Hospital. At the Phipps Clinic he held the Henderson research scholarship in psychiatry for two years until he left for the famous Burghoelzli Clinic in Switzerland to study under Hans W. Meier, the successor of Eugene Bleuler, another man who had significantly influenced psychiatric thinking.

In Switzerland, Cameron met the principal psychiatrist of the province of Manitoba, A. T. Mathers, who convinced the young Scot to come to Manitoba. This would seem to be a rather curious choice for an aspiring psychiatrist, since the prairie heartland of Canada was most certainly not in the forefront of psychiatry in the 1920s. Whatever his reason for going, however, Cameron had a successful career in Manitoba. While in charge of the admitting unit of the provincial mental hospital in Brandon, he organized the mental health services in the western part of the province. He developed a network of ten clinics in Brandon and outlying areas that was the forerunner of the community mental health models of the 1960s. At the same time, he pursued clinical research and contributed to scientific literature.

In 1936, he moved to Massachusetts to become director of the research division at Worcester State Hospital, and from 1939 to 1943 he was professor of neurology and psychiatry at Albany Medical College in Albany, New York, and at the Russell Sage School of Nursing, also in the Albany area. During those years, Cameron began to expand on his thoughts about the interrelationships of mind and body, and developed a reputation as a psychiatrist who could bridge the gap between the organic, structural neurologists, and the psychiatrists whose knowledge of anatomy was limited to maps of the mind as opposed to maps of the brain. He also became noted as a thoughtful teacher.

Cameron's early papers are illustrative of the biological descriptive psychiatry of the time—especially of the British and European schools. Psychiatry was very much modeled on a disease concept of mental disturbance. Papers in the literature focused on describing in detail the behavioral syndromes and on offering hypotheses about the psychological mechanisms that might underlie the disorders. In his own writings, Cameron wrote about schizophrenia, its phenomenology and treatment, and about psychotic syndromes that are caused by physical changes in the brain. Several papers reveal the beginnings of Cameron's lifelong interest in memory. Cameron was fascinated by the question of how memories are formed: Where in the brain does this take place? What changes occur during this process? And what biological reactions permit us to recall those memories we do store? His early work also describes his nascent interest in the problems of aging, especially the psychoses associated with changes in the brain.

In 1936, Cameron published his first book, *Objective and Experimental Psychiatry*. It introduced his lifelong belief that psychiatry should strive to approach the study of human behavior in a rigorous, scientific fashion. Clearly rooted in biology, his theories of behavior stressed the unity of the organism with the environment. Throughout the text, emphasis is placed on the experimental method and research design. Thus we see "an essential aspect of the true experiment is that one should test one's theory of the dynamics of the experiment by comparing the actual result with the predicted result." He laments: "Unfortunately, it cannot be claimed for psychiatry that the observational method has ever approached this degree of technical accuracy." Cameron, the young psychiatrist, thus followed the tradition of clinical psychiatry and charted his course as a firm adherent of the scientific method.

In 1943 he was invited to McGill University in Montreal at the urgings of the world-famous neurosurgeon, Wilder Penfield. There, with a grant from the Rockefeller Foundation, money from J. D. McConnell of the *Montreal Star*, and a gift of the mansion of Sir Hugh Allan on Mount Royal, the Allan Memorial Institute was founded. For the next twenty-one years, Cameron's vision, determination, and adroit political maneuvering led to the astounding growth of the Institute. Psychiatrists were recruited from Europe and around the world to build a program of unparalleled scope. Although committed to a biological understanding of psychiatry, Cameron brought in psychoanalysts, social psychiatrists, and biologists. He also developed a network of psychiatric services for Montreal. During these years, Cameron was at his peak, extending his reputation worldwide.

Cameron's growing reputation was evident by 1945, when he was one of three North American psychiatrists invited to Nuremberg to evaluate Rudolph Hess. This was an opportunity for him to represent the new Canadian psychiatry, to draw attention to his rapidly evolving institute in Montreal, and to reinforce his stature in the profession. He was among a select group—Krasnushkin, Sepp, and Kurshakov of the Soviet Union; Lord Moran, Rees, and Riddoch from England; Lewis, Schroeder, and himself from North America; and Professor Delay from France. Yet the honor he was accorded in being invited to Nuremberg grew out of an abyss of horror. The hours of daily testimony told of the millions of people destroyed by an evil unparalleled in history. In Germany, Cameron could hear at first hand how a nation could corrupt itself; he could begin to appreciate the social forces that could mold a culture into a killing machine. Germany was a laboratory in which the issues of authority, powerlessness, individual motivation, and behavior could be examined by behavioral and social scientists—if they could overcome their disgust.

The commission was asked to answer two questions about Hess. First, was he sufficiently competent to plead to the charge? Second, was he sane or not? More specifically, did he have sufficient intellect to comprehend what was taking place and to defend himself? Could he challenge a witness? And could he understand the evidence that would be presented? Hess had made two suicide attempts; he was also reported to have shown delusions of persecution and other manifestations of paranoia and to have been affected by amnesia for significant periods of his life. Given all of this, the request for evaluation seemed reasonable and challenging, and Cameron loved a challenge. Following examinations of Hess on November 15 and 19, 1945, and the perusal of a great deal of data, the three psychiatrists from North America and the one from France concluded that Rudolf Hess "is not insane at the present time in the strict sense of the word." He ultimately was sentenced to life in prison.

Seven months prior to serving as a consultant to the International Military Tribunals at Nuremberg, Cameron had written a paper entitled "The Social Reorganization of Germany." In this work, he examined the interaction between the culture of Germany and the character patterns of individuals. His thesis focused on the need for a major "transformation of the existing cultural organization" in the postwar period. He talked about such characteristics of German culture as the need for status, the worship of order and regimentation, authoritarian leadership, and the fear of other countries. He speculated that, thirty years in the future, the adolescents of the Third Reich would represent the greatest threat to world peace. The paper suggested both short- and long-term interventions, but the overall proposal focused on the need to destroy the social organization that had repeatedly given birth to such fearsome aggression. He emphasized the need for a world order, and clearly he was struggling to understand how forces outside the individual could engulf so many in such horror.

Six weeks after his return from Nuremberg, he tried to put some of his thoughts about the experience into words. In a paper entitled "Nuremberg and Its Significance," Cameron noted that the trials were immensely important and useful for three reasons: the first was the reestablishment of justice in Europe; the second was the confrontation of the German people with the facts of the atrocities committed during the war; and the third lay in the revelations to the world that all this had occurred. He concluded:

> It is not simply against future conspiracies of evil men which we have to guard ourselves but it is against ourselves, against weaknesses and faults in our own social order, in our own ways of living against which we have to be on continual guard.

He went on to present the need for more knowledge concerning the interactions between human beings and the dangers that they present to each other. His conclusion was that social and behavioral scientists must concern themselves not only with individuals, but with the ways in which they function in society. His goal was to destroy "dangerous and out-dated concepts of human relations" before these could hurt society. In a radio talk six months later, he again expressed his concern that, in all segments of our society, there were people in authority who infect the rest of us with "perilously misleading beliefs concerning human beings"; he gave the example of those "bow and arrow minds" who could have access to atomic power. The future lay in the direction of the knowledge that could be gained from psychology, sociology, and psychiatry—knowledge that he felt must override the resistance of outdated concepts. He saw the social and behavioral scientists as the planners of the social systems of our society. In addition, he saw the need for a more united world and embraced the concept of the United Nations.

In his broad thinking, he did not differ significantly from many who were trying to conceive of a world where the nightmare of Nazism could never again emerge. However, he was a psychiatrist, a student of human behavior, and he was imbued with a fervor about what he thought the relatively young science of psychiatry could offer the world. Over time, his writings began to reflect a sense that the world was made up of the strong and the weak, the latter being those with anxieties or insecurities. The strong would need to protect others from these people; they could not be allowed to influence children. Some of the weak he called "dangerous men and women." Thus, the lesson that this psychiatrist took from Nuremberg was the need to protect society from those who could bring it once more to chaos; these people would need to be identified and their roles in society evaluated. Behavioral scientists were in an excellent position to undertake this task. In his zeal for a new world order where chaos was controlled, Cameron carried within him the potential for repeating the mistakes of the past.

As he hit his stride in the late 1940s and early 1950s, Cameron began to broaden his areas of interest. His work in memory and aging continued, as seen in a book called *Remembering* and in papers on experimental procedures to improve memory using RNA (ribonucleic acid). In addition, further descriptions of clinical states such as anxiety, depression, and schizophrenia demonstrated his continued commitment to clinical psychiatry. He began to write about teaching psychiatry, about the organization of clinical services, and about psychotherapy.

At the same time, his interest in social psychiatry became increasingly apparent. Social psychiatry is an area that examines the roles of interpersonal interaction, family, community, and culture in the genesis and amelioration of emotional disturbance. Cameron's work in the field took several forms. He was the first psychiatrist to introduce the concept of the day hospital—a place for patients to receive treatment during the day and to return to their families at night. He explored the place of psychiatric units in general hospitals and strongly encouraged psychiatric treatment that examined both the social and "intrapsychic" (psychological) factors of illness. Questioning the usefulness of Freud's concepts, he noted that "it is doubtful whether [the concept of the unconscious] should be continued since it too imposes many limitations upon our thinking. . . ." With his social science perspective, he raised new questions:

> We can see that what we have been dealing with is the way in which human activity expresses itself in terms of our culture. . . . [We must then consider] what is the most effective form of personality development and what modifications in our cultural pattern must be brought about to permit such personality development.

Cameron began to explore the importance of work to the individual by examining the psychological characteristics of work and the relation of human behavior to industry.

A careful examination of Cameron's activities and writings during these years reveals his central preoccupation. First, Cameron strongly believed in a biological basis for most severe psychopathology, and so, by description and experimentation on memory, he hoped to understand the determinants of severe psychopathology. Second, he felt that Freud had produced a theory that served only to narrow the horizons of psychiatry—a theory that should be discarded. He was, however, to remain so ambivalent about Freud that, although he never became a psychoanalyst, he was to use Freudian conceptions of development in a somewhat idiosyncratic way as a basis for understanding the motivations of his patients. Third, the early influence of Adolph Meyer made him begin to examine those external influences on thinking and behavior that might at times interact with biology to produce or ameliorate illness.

Cameron's work over the late 1940s and early 1950s also revealed a growing interest in the role of psychiatry as an agent of social change. The origins of this interest appear to lie in Cameron's experiences at the war crimes trials in Nuremberg. As part of the multinational team of psychiatrists, Cameron actively participated in considering the impact of the holocaust. In 1946, in a paper titled "Frontiers of Social Psychiatry," Cameron for the first time used the case of Nazi Germany as an example of a society that poisoned the minds of its citizens through the propagation of anxiety. His startling conclusion was that social psychiatry must contribute to developing methods of social control over its citizens in order to direct "the transmission of attitudes, beliefs, and ways of managing life." He expressed this authoritarian perspective in a series of remarkable statements:

> We now recognize that the transmission to children, and also to people at all ages[,] of beliefs, attitudes, and customs which produce unnecessary anxiety, guilt, feelings of inadequacy and hostility, must come to an end as a matter of public health and individual well-being. We have recognized that many of these damaging ways of being are transmitted by parents who themselves suffer from them. We also recognize the part played by social institutions interested in perpetuating themselves.

He suggested that psychiatry must be "inventive" and determine "rapid ways of building up new attitudes for social control without crippling guilt." He then noted that children have "certain psychological rights" which include the right "to protection against indoctrination with damaging, outmoded attitudes, against the implantation of taboos and inhibitions" by their parents. His proposal was startling:

> All of us have seen the transmission down the generations of insecurity, chronic anxiety, frigidity, feelings of inadequacy. We have at present no means whatsoever of stopping this. It could be stopped, however, by remodelling and expanding our present concepts of suitability for marriage, of quarantine of individuals suffering from diseases likely to spread to others.

In the book *Life Is for Living*, published in 1948 for a general audience, Cameron further expanded on the concept of determining who should have children and who should hold positions of authority. He was quite concerned about people who had been influenced by the Nazis:

> If we can succeed in inventing means of changing their attitudes and beliefs, we shall find ourselves in possession of measures which, if wisely used, may be employed in freeing

ourselves from attitudes and beliefs in other fields which have greatly contributed to the instability of our period by their propensity for holding up progress.

In another paper, Cameron discussed the concept of contagion as related to psychological happenings. Although society had established sanctions against the spread of infectious diseases, this had not occurred with respect to chronic anxiety. He warned that people afflicted with this disorder could become "potentially spreading" liabilities who might transmit their anxiety to others. Similarly, in an undated talk that appears to have been given in the late 1940s, Cameron presented a set of ideas which are quite unusual. The talk was titled "Dangerous Men and Women," and in it he described various personality types that he felt were of significant danger to society. These individuals were seen as dangerous to their friends and colleagues, and destructive to their children.

The first type he pointed to was the passive personality—a man who "is afraid to say what he really thinks. . . . he will stand [for] anything, and stands for nothing; he was born in Munich—he is the eternal compromiser and his spiritual food is appeasement." The second he termed the possessive type; these people are filled with jealousy and demand utmost loyalty. Their danger is to those who are closest to them; their effect on children can be devastating. The third category was the insecure man: "They are the driven crowd that makes the army of the authoritarian overlord; they are the stuffing of conservatism. . . . mediocrity is their god. They fear the stranger, they fear the new idea; they are afraid to live, and scared to die." These people try hard to conform to the dictates of society—a world of strict right and wrong that is manipulated by power groups to keep the insecure under control and dependent, and a danger. Science must contribute to changing the world in such a way as to release these weak people from the fears that keep them so miserable. The last personality, the psychopath, presents the greatest danger at times of political upheaval; this was the type that entered the Gestapo.

Cameron was caught up in trying to make the world a

better place. In order to do this, political systems had to be watched, and those personalities that had allowed Nazism to flourish needed to be controlled. "Get it understood how dangerous these damaged, sick personalities are to ourselves—and above all, to our children, whose traits are taking form—and we shall find ways to put an end to them," Cameron wrote. It is surprising to hear the denigration by a psychiatrist of people who are crippled by emotional handicaps. They are not presented with concern or understanding, but are rather described as a force to be reckoned with by society. Thus, Cameron's solution to the ills of society was simple: Experts should decide who can parent and who should govern. These experts must develop methods of forcefully changing attitudes and beliefs.

By the mid-1950s, Ewen Cameron had reached the top of his field. He was professor of psychiatry at McGill University, psychiatrist-in-chief of the Royal Victoria Hospital, and director of the Allan Memorial Institute of Psychiatry. Within a short time he was elected president of the American Psychiatric Association, the Quebec Psychiatric Association, the Canadian Psychiatric Association, the World Psychiatric Association, the American Psychopathological Association, and the Society of Biological Psychiatry. In fact, one of his colleagues said, only partially in jest, "We have run out of presidencies to give him. We shall now have to form another association for him." Thanks to the network of professional relationships he had created, the Allan Memorial Institute was catapulted within a short space of time to the position of one of the foremost institutions for psychiatric research and clinical treatment in the world.

But what of those who knew Ewen Cameron personally? It is surprising, years later, to hear the comments of those who worked with him. A mixture of admiration and awe combined with fear appears in many of the comments. Thus, one of his colleagues notes that he was "a very decisive person, [a] really impressive man" who "created his own way of thinking." He goes on, however, to remark that "anyone working with him was really under him. We were just little kids." D. O. Hebb, one of the world's foremost psychologists, was chairman of the Department of Psychology at McGill at that time. He commented during an interview that Cameron had achieved eminence primarily on the basis of his ability to function well in the political arena. Concerning his experimental work, Hebb said that Cameron "didn't have the faintest notion of how to go about doing experiments or doing research. But he thought he did." In a later interview, given to film makers Ron Blumer, my oldest friend, and his wife, Muffie Meyer, the week before Hebb died, he commented: "He [Cameron] wasn't so much driven with wanting to know; he was driven with wanting to be important—to make that breakthrough. It made him a bad scientist." It is also said of Cameron that he could fall for a new idea even if it were unscientific. His zeal to transcend the boundaries of psychiatric knowledge could blur his ability to see the limitations of new directions; his impatience could make the scientific method seem too slow or unimportant.

Cameron was seen as a hard worker and brilliant organizer. But he was also seen as distant and unfriendly, "not a cocktail party man." Another of his colleagues told an anecdote that is particularly revealing:

> Nobody was close to him. He never accepted an invitation to any party of any staff member, or invited anyone to his home. . . . I had a tragedy during this point . . . but Cameron didn't say anything to me. When I left, I said that it had [been] very intellectually stimulating to work with you, but you are impersonal. He said, "No, I'm not impersonal. I know what you went through. I kept an eye on you."

A resident in training at the time notes that the residents were all afraid of him, of his power, and yet "he had never done anything bad to anyone." It is the sense of his absolute power that permeates all the comments about Dr. Cameron—the odd combination of respect tinged with fear. Another of his residents remarked, "If I wanted to stay in Montreal, it would have been wise for me to accept his frame of reference."

Two of Cameron's junior colleagues who are now preeminent in the field have described their sense of powerlessness in the face of his ability to control their destinies. One of these men noted Cameron's "arrogance, detachment, and condescending attitude." He further revealed that some of the scientists at the Allan Memorial were embarrassed at research meetings because of the jokes around Cameron's citing his own work so much in his research papers. The implication is that Dr. Cameron had a profound need to see himself as a great scientist and innovator. It was the feeling of this colleague that Cameron was "turned off" by such fundamental principles of scientific methodology as the use of control subjects, a method of experimentation in which a group of similar subjects is not given the treatment and then compared to the group where the intervention has been applied. Cameron, the colleague noted, would see rigorous research methods as "bureaucratic nonsense." This colleague felt that Cameron needed to have "yes-men" around him; perhaps he "was dimly aware of his shortcomings."

The second of these colleagues described Cameron as "a man of integrity, if you could tap into it." He saw his old chief as a "great individualist . . . charismatic, and kind." Yet he also remembers that Cameron had very rigid ideas about career development. As an example, he cites Cameron's warning to him not to publish a certain paper because such a piece would "only be appropriate for psychiatrists in the fifth decade of life." He was told that he would do himself "incalculable harm" if he persisted. Another memory that stood out for this man was a statement that Cameron made about the future of a younger colleague who had displeased him. Promotion and assistance was not going to be forthcoming from the "professor"; Cameron said, "Let him sit under a cold water spout," as he abandoned him to his fate.

It is interesting to consider what Cameron thought about his tenure as director of the Institute. Fortunately, he began to record his thoughts on this subject in 1964 when he began to work on a book about medical institutes. He was interested in writing about how such institutions develop and what transpires in their evolution. His ideas about the role of a director are forceful and clear: "He is an integrator . . . he is the person who must hold the organization together. You cannot lead from somewhere halfway back. . . .

He must undoubtedly be somebody who is good at something . . . [with] a measure of excellence." He wrote that it had been an honor and a valuable opportunity for him to serve as director of the Allan and to be a part of a great university. Most important, he described his joy and pride at being a part of the development of psychiatry—"to have worked in a field which encompasses the whole of man . . . and beyond that to have challenged to seek out those changes in his brain, in his chemistry, and in his very structure which might disturb him in his littlest and in his greatest dealings with himself and his world."

Ewen Cameron appears to have been a man for whom science was a deity; he was single-minded in his pursuit of his version of truth. Relationships paled in importance, except, perhaps, those with his wife and four children. One is left with the picture of a man whose power and drive provoked fear and respect, but whose own quest for understanding was of such intensity that all else was simply irrelevant.

Cameron became an American citizen in 1942 and never sought to obtain Canadian citizenship. As Quebec entered the "quiet revolution" of the 1960s and French-Canadians increasingly clamored for greater recognition of their language and culture, Cameron became increasingly disaffected with the tide of change. In 1964 he left Montreal to return to Albany as director of the Psychiatry and Aging Research Laboratory at the Veterans Administration Hospital and at Albany Medical College.

It would appear that several factors contributed to Cameron's move to Albany. Some of his colleagues whom I interviewed attribute most of the impetus for the departure to Cameron's inability to reconcile himself to the French fact of life in Quebec. First, problems were beginning to emerge between Cameron and those in power in Quebec City, especially with those officials involved in the administration of health grants. Second, Cameron's relationship with Wilder Penfield, the eminent director of the Montreal Neurological Institute, had cooled rapidly over the years. While Penfield had been instrumental in recruiting Cameron to McGill, he had not reckoned on Cameron's independent ways. Whether their differences were political, philosophical, or scientific is not clear; what is known, however, is that Cameron no longer enjoyed the support of the influential neurosurgeon. Lastly, it would appear that Cameron's work in psychic driving must have become increasingly controversial. This is suggested by the fact that Robert Cleghorn, Cameron's successor, put an end to depatterning at the Allan Memorial Institute almost as soon as Cameron had departed. In addition, he asked two of his colleagues to carry out a study designed to evaluate the effects of intensive ECT, and ordered one of Cameron's adherents to discontinue this line of "treatment." The work to which Cameron had devoted the last ten years of his professional life came to an abrupt end.

Cameron, himself, described his reason for leaving in a letter that he wrote in May 1964 to Dr. C. F. Cyril James, the former principal of McGill University. In that letter, Cameron announces his intention to leave in August and notes, "My reasons are very difficult to follow even for myself." He then states that twenty-one years is a long time to be doing the same thing and that it is time to move on. He also notes that, at sixty-two years of age, he had only three more years to be director, after which he would have had to "be on the sidelines which I should not like." At Albany, he could work as long as he was able.

During the years following his departure from McGill, Cameron remained active in the profession. He returned to an early interest by continuing his examination of memory and the treatment of memory loss in the elderly. His last major work was published posthumously in 1968. Entitled *Psychotherapy in Action*, it represents a synthesis of his ideas concerning what therapy does, and in many ways is an updated version of his earlier book, *General Psychotherapy: Dynamics and Procedures*.

Ewen Cameron died on September 9, 1967, by which time he had written one hundred and fifty-four scientific papers and five books. He died of a massive heart attack at the top of a mountain in the Adirondacks in New York State after conquering the peak with his youngest son. He had long expressed a desire to climb this mountain, to be on top—truly a metaphor for his life.

Cameron was a man of enormous energy and determination. He was also a visionary; he saw a role for his profession in the post-war world, and he seized every opportunity to provide psychiatry with a status that would allow it to be influential in the political and social cross-currents of the time. Although he claimed that his roots lay in biology, and in social and behavioral science, he was not a truly successful researcher in any of these areas of knowledge. As a clinician, he was either loved or hated; as a teacher, he was both revered and feared; as a man, few were able to penetrate the veneer of Scottish taciturnity; none whom I am aware of counted him as a close friend.

Cameron, whether through messianic zeal, misguided adventurism, or misplaced patriotism, participated in the covert work of the CIA. He used unknowing patients for mind-control experimentation and, in so doing, made a mockery of the doctor-patient relationship. And yet, this same man was described as follows in a biographical sketch in 1953 at the time of his presidential address to the American Psychiatric Association:

> His is an attitude not of an individualist who seeks to impress his own personal drives on his contemporaries, but rather of a public servant (so typical of the old-fashioned and straightforward Anglo-Saxon) who lives the major trends of his time in unison with and for the community he lives in, without drooping to become a dull conformist.

Ewen Cameron was a man of extremes—taciturn and kind, grandiose and callous—and he remains today a paradox, an enigma.

This was my father's doctor.

8

The Experiment

The tune plays in my mind at times. Like some long-forgotten love song it returns, beguiling and seducing me into remembrance. The thoughts evoked are not the sweet memories of a lost lover, nor the gentle reminiscences of youthful escape. Over and over I hear the refrain:

> *Mares eat oats and does eat oats*
> *And little lambs eat ivy. . . .*

Around and around in my head, I hear his voice, my father's voice, singing tunelessly. From one end of the house to the other he paces; "Mares eat oats . . . maresy dotes . . . doesy doats. . . ." Will it ever end? I feel at a loss; I cannot fathom the anxiety that he feels. Tonight he is going to the hospital and treatment will make him well. "Dr. Cameron is a good doctor," my mother says, "Daddy will be home very soon." Reassured, I leave for school.

Thirty years later, it is the summer of 1986. I stand at the bottom of the hill and look at the old gray building, Ravenscrag—the Allan Memorial Institute. It seems innocent enough; one of Montreal's old stone mansions commanding a magnificent view on the mountain overlooking the St.

Lawrence River. I am on a quest for knowledge, greedily consuming every scrap of information that I can find. Who was Cameron? What did he do in the sleep rooms? Who understands what happened? Who will talk to me?

Today, I will return to the Allan for the first time since medical school. I will walk through those doors and into the same lobby that forms the backdrop of memory. This morning I will return to see a former colleague of Ewen Cameron and I will ask questions. As I walk up the road, the tune begins to play, "Maresy doats and doesy doats." The tempo quickens and my anxiety rises as I reach the main entrance. I must learn the truth. What manner of experiment took place here? Why was my father chosen? I enter the doors drenched with sweat. I live in the past and in the present. Can I shut the music off? Can I bury the dead?

The student arrives to learn the experiment.

Throughout his long career, Ewen Cameron was interested in physical methods (chemical or electrical) that could be either used to treat severely disturbed people or utilized in psychotherapy to diminish a patient's defenses. Such "disinhibition" would then give the therapist access to memories and feelings that the patient would normally be unable to express. In his first book, Cameron describes the use of such drugs as mescaline, Benzedrine, caffeine, alcohol, sodium amytal, cocaine, and others for these purposes.

Cameron's orientation to physical methods of treatment was a reflection of the evolution of psychiatry during the early part of this century. Historically, there were increasing attempts to control the symptoms of major psychiatric disturbance with treatments that would work directly on the brain and perhaps influence behavioral pathways. Much of this work was done in the major European centers, but gradually the same approaches were explored in the United States as well. Such treatments included baths and wrapping in sheets, insulin shock treatment, lobotomy, and electroconvulsive therapy. Manfred Sakel, in 1928, developed the insulin coma treatment that was used for many years to control the excited states of severely psychotic patients. In 1935, Egas Moniz and Almeida Lima carried out the first lobotomies. This operation involved the cutting of fibers from an area of the brain that appeared to be responsible for emotion. Emotional responses were then changed so that tensions would not accumulate and result in behavioral disorder.

In 1938, U. Cerletti and L. Bini in Italy developed the process of electroconvulsive therapy (ECT). It had been noted that epilepsy and schizophrenia rarely occurred in the same patient and that a seizure would often clear symptoms of psychosis. The use of ECT was thus an attempt to achieve the effects resulting from insulin coma but with fewer complications. The technique involved the passage of a current of 70 to 130 volts through the brain for 0.1 to 0.5 seconds. A generalized seizure was necessary, so that if this did not occur during the first attempt, the ECT treatment could be repeated at a higher voltage for a longer period. ECT was generally given once a day. As time passed, combinations of techniques were used, such as insulin coma with ECT. Lastly, chemical agents that would induce seizures were tried.

Today, many of these physical procedures appear almost barbaric, but we should remember that in the 1930s and 1940s antipsychotic medications were not yet available. Asylums were filled with men and women who shouted and cried incessantly, who fought and killed, who curled up in corners and never talked again. Psychiatrists were faced with attempting to help these people and sought cures wherever they could find them. During the first half of this century, the physical procedures were the treatment of choice. However, with increased knowledge and the appearance of the first antipsychotic drug, chlorpromazine (Thorazine), psychiatry moved rapidly away from these extreme treatments. The most severely disturbed patients could then be discharged from the hospitals, no longer having to face the dangers of insulin coma or the irreversible brain damage of lobotomies. The new drugs were to bring their own dangers, such as neurological damage, but initially they were filled with promise for those whose lives were filled with torment.

At the same time that these physical methods of treatment were evolving, psychiatry was developing in an entirely different direction. Following the discoveries of Sigmund Freud, therapists and theorists built upon or modified his work to elucidate the psychodynamic understanding of the personality. Freud, Jung, and their disciples evolved a model of understanding and a method of treatment (psychoanalysis) that was long and expensive, had mixed results, and appeared to be useful only for certain types of patients. However, psychological theories of human behavior increasingly dominated psychiatric thinking, and by the 1950s psychoanalysts occupied the chairmanships of most of the major departments of psychiatry in the United States.

In England and Europe, meanwhile, work continued on organic treatments for psychosis and depression, and by 1952 the first psychoactive drugs were introduced—the first being chlorpromazine. In 1948 the English psychiatrists L. E. M. Page and R. J. Russell reported for the first time their use of a particularly intensive form of electroconvulsive therapy. Treatment consisted of an initial stimulus of 150 volts for one second, followed by five shocks of 100 volts during the primary convulsion. These were usually given once a day, occasionally twice daily in the most severe cases. It was suggested that their use was most effective in treating schizophrenia, psychotic depression, and paranoid psychosis. By 1953 Page and Russell had given this treatment to 3,500 individuals and had increased the number of secondary shocks from five to a range of seven to ten. They gave each patient eight to fifteen ECTs with an average of three or four treatments for depression. These English physicians appeared to be following the hypothesis that if a little bit of electricity was helpful, a great deal would be even better. It is true that they were attempting to treat virtually hopeless people, but some of these physicians' reservations about the extreme methods are evident in their concern that no patient should ever see or hear another patient receiving treatment.

In the United States, this approach was adopted in some centers for the treatment of cases of schizophrenia that were resistant to all other therapies. One investigator described a process that involved regressing patients to the level of four-year-olds—wetting, soiling, and unable to care for themselves. Another investigator worried about the possibility of permanent brain damage, but nevertheless increased applications from twenty-eight to sixty-five shock treatments given three times a day, seven days a week. This group of psychiatrists described their regressed patients as confused and disoriented, with no memory or a lack of verbal spontaneity; they had slurred speech or were completely mute, and were apathetic, incontinent, and unable to swallow—they required feeding through a nasogastric tube. They showed many signs of neurological impairment while in this state, including primitive reflexes that are usually seen only in newborn infants. After seven to ten days, the patients gradually emerged from this state with a reversal of the regressive process. Although the physicians noted that minimal complications occurred, the patients suffered a permanent amnesia for the two to three months prior to treatment. Gradual improvement was observed over five years. These treatments were seen by most of the investigators as a treatment of last resort. When all else had failed, these extreme forms of treatment could be tried. The final resort was lobotomy.

In 1955, Hassan Azima at the Allan Memorial Institute adapted a treatment that had been developed in the Soviet Union, the so-called "sleep treatment." This method consisted of the administration of a mixture of Thorazine and barbiturates on a continual basis so as to provoke a sleep pattern as similar as possible to normal sleep. Patients would thus sleep twenty to twenty-two hours daily for weeks. Like ECTs, drug-induced sleep treatment was seen as appropriate only for extreme cases.

In the midst of these developments, Ewen Cameron began to evolve a series of ideas designed to change behavior. He had little patience for the kind of psychotherapy espoused by his analytic colleagues; he felt that the process was too long and did not adequately deal with very ill people. From his writings, it appears that his dream was to find a way of changing long-standing maladaptive or dysfunctional personality patterns quickly, thus introducing "more healthy" behavior without the need for psychoanalysis.

In 1950, a paper appeared that described an attempt to

directly "reorient behavior patterns" through the use of "deep narcosis." This paper clearly influenced Cameron's work for the next fifteen years.

The theory was as follows: the ways in which people behave are determined by some sort of nervous system arrangements in the brain. Since psychotherapy can change behavior, the neural arrangements must be reversible. The authors wondered whether the behavior patterns of adults could be erased by a physiologic process that attacked neural patterns. Could adults be made theoretically patternless? Could they be returned to a state of neurologic and psychologic infancy for a short period, and then could new patterns of behavior be introduced? Using a barbiturate (sodium amytal), these investigators induced a state of "clinical coma" in their patients and read to them prepared scripts taken from their lives. They were not particularly successful, but Cameron chose their experiments as the starting point for the evolution of his theories concerning rapid behavior and attitude change.

In 1956, in a paper titled "Psychic Driving," Cameron reported for the first time on a technique that he had been developing since 1953. He noted that, if patients were made to listen to recorded playback of emotionally laden material that they had reported to the therapist, this could be a "gateway through which we might pass to a new field of psychotherapeutic methods." The procedure required the patients to listen to these tape recordings for long periods of time. He called the technique "driving" and described two forms: the first, autopsychic driving, where patients listened to their own voices; the second, heteropsychic driving, where the recording was based on emotional material suggested by the patients, but interpreted by others. The purpose of the approach was to penetrate the patient's psychological defenses, to bring out conflict-laden thoughts and feelings that the patient would not normally reveal, and to set up what Cameron termed a "dynamic implant"—a focus in the brain of "increased reactivity" that would continue to produce hitherto repressed material.

Initially, the procedure was carried out for thirty minutes once a week, but gradually the length of exposure and frequency were dramatically increased. He described the attempts of his research group to find better ways of delivering the messages and of preparing the patients to receive them—thus, pillow and ceiling microphones, working variations on the message with different voices and styles, and role-playing. He also introduced for the first time the need to disinhibit the patients so as to lower the defenses and allow the patient to hear the material. Techniques to facilitate this result included the use of sodium amytal, stimulant drugs (amphetamines), prolonged sleep with driving ten to twenty hours a day for ten to fifteen days, and, most startling, placing patients in prolonged psychological isolation. This involved placing patients in a dark room, covering their eyes with goggles, reducing auditory intake, and preventing them from touching their bodies. Lastly, Cameron described the use of LSD to produce disinhibition. He told how patients reacted and noted that the responses ranged from recognition of the conflict to blocking, avoiding, rejecting, and otherwise attempting to defend against hearing the material. One patient, he noted, had become psychotic.

In a second paper, delivered in 1957, Cameron elaborated on his theory of the "dynamic implant." He postulated that, in response to a "driving" or "cue" statement, a response takes place in the brain that sensitizes the patient to the suggested issues. Consequently, the patient continues to be aware of the concerns and all the associated conflicts of the driving statement for an ongoing period of time. He describes one patient's response to the technique. At the end of five minutes:

> "It makes me nervous, you'd better stop it . . . it makes me feel bad." . . . She was now restless and anxious and very different from the gay person she had been when she came at the beginning of the hour. At eight minutes, "Doctor, doctor. I've had enough, please stop it." Holds head. Nine minutes, "That's enough. It makes me nervous to hear that." Ten minutes, "Why don't you stop it, doctor. I've heard enough. It is always the same."

Cameron reassured his audience that in two years of using this technique with more than one hundred patients, there had been only one persisting trauma. Yet the patient's dialogue that is reported above occurs after only ten minutes of driving on one occasion; what would happen after hours of exposure on multiple occasions? Cameron went on to refine his technique; he began to use headphones so that the voices would sound as though they came from inside the patient's head. He then developed filtered recordings with the emphasis on high notes or low, at high or low volume. He could also space or repeat parts of the message and use echoes. Ultimately, multiple voices were used.

What made this approach unique was that Cameron was combining physical methods with his version of psychotherapy. What further differentiated the method was its use of techniques to break down the patient's defenses and, when the patient was most vulnerable, to expose this man or woman to hours of repetition of a painful message. This had never been attempted in any psychiatric institution. In addition, in his attempts to force the patients to change, Cameron went further with these extreme methods than had ever been reported. Worse, these profoundly intrusive procedures were applied to patients who were not severely disturbed. Under Cameron, what was previously last-stage intervention rapidly became front-line treatment.

By 1960, Cameron and his colleagues had considerably refined the driving technique, which he also termed "ultraconceptual communication." The refinements were based primarily on methods of breaking down the patient's resistance to change. Driving now consisted of very long periods of exposure to recorded messages—sixteen hours a day for twenty to thirty days. The patients were given a drug called Sernyl [1-(1-phenylcyclohexyl)piperidine monohydrochloride], or PCP, to "block sensory input and produce underactivity." This drug, which was designed as an anesthetic for animals, produces acute psychotic episodes and even the danger of chronic psychosis in humans. Thorazine was added to the regimen to enhance the effect and control the anxiety that was secondary to the Sernyl. This produced a "passive receptive state with a heightened awareness of the verbal signals." Intensive ECT was added for more resistant patients, and patients also received electroshock at the end of the repetition cycle of recorded messages. These modifications to the original design were described as part of a treatment approach for "chronic psychoneurotic patients."

Such extreme physical procedures represented a massive departure from the accepted psychodynamic methods for overcoming resistance and eliciting the hidden thoughts, feelings, and memories of neurotic patients. Standard psychotherapy of the kind that had evolved over the first fifty years of this century was based upon a relationship between patient and therapist that slowly develops out of trust. As the relationship progresses, the patient gradually opens up and reveals to the physician the many secrets and fantasies that he hides from the world. At the same time, a unique relationship emerges that is called "transference." This involves the development of feelings toward the therapist that are a reflection of earlier feelings that the patient had toward significant figures in his life, usually parents. An understanding of these "transferred" feelings underlies the basis of the psychotherapy. This process had been discovered by Freud and then refined, both by his disciples and by those who took different paths over the years. It requires patience on the part of the therapist and an ability to tolerate the patient's symptoms.

Cameron did not have either the patience or the ability to accept the fact that symptom relief for certain kinds of patients may take a significant time. Consequently, at the Allan Memorial Institute, patients who were not severely disturbed did not receive a cautious and careful therapy; instead they were subjected to extreme physical procedures designed to force an entry into their minds by breaking down their defenses. Change was seen as capitulation to a bombardment with emotion-laden verbal messages. The approach appears to be simplistic, but Cameron never questioned the efficacy of his technique. He noted that "reorganization of the personality could be brought about without the necessity of solving conflicts or abreaction, or reliving past experiences." The psychic driving would result in the direct building of new personality traits; older ones would remain but be put out of circuit. Clearly, as the work progressed, increased effort was put into immobilizing the individuals, forcing them to attend to increasingly powerful recordings and breaking down their natural ability to fight off the intrusive messages. Chillingly, he comments: "Obviously, what has been achieved with respect to psychoneurotic patients can be extended to any field in which there is malfunction of the personality, *whether within the area of psychiatry or not.*" One can only wonder whether this comment is an allusion to the forced conversions or brainwashing techniques of the Chinese Communists that were being described both in the news media and in literature during the early 1950s.

The process whereby patients were immobilized, rendered intellectually helpless, and prevented from utilizing the usual defenses was developed into a procedure that Cameron called "depatterning." He felt that, if he could destroy the ongoing patterns of behavior by disruption of the brain pathways, he could then start with a clean slate—a *tabula rasa.* He wrote in 1958 that the intent of depatterning was to treat severely disturbed individuals (schizophrenics) in this manner, and he described three formats: intensive ECT at least twice a day, sleep treatment and intensive ECT, and sleep alone. One depatterning format that he outlined was as follows: sleep twenty to twenty-two hours a day maintained by Thorazine and a combination of barbiturates (Seconal, pentobarbital, phenobarbital). During this time, the patient was wakened three times a day for meals and toilet. Solid food was given the first week, then semisolid, and insulin was given before every meal. After ten days of sleep, Page-Russell shock treatments were given to produce complete depatterning between thirty to sixty days after thirty intensified shock treatments. The ECTs were then continued at the rate of three a week.

A major goal of this program was to produce "differential amnesia." Cameron believed that if one could totally wipe out memory, on its return pathological patterns would be much less readily recalled to memory than the normal ones. Although he initially reported that twenty to thirty ECTs were usual, he noted that many patients received considerably more; in fact, he states that the range was twenty-three to one hundred and fifty, with an average of sixty-six. There was also a hint that less severely ill patients were being treated in this way.

Depatterning was a three-stage process in which patients lost track progressively of time and space. It was a disturbance of memory so massive that it could not be measured, and this was Cameron's attempt to clarify the infantile regression that had earlier been described in intensive shock treatment. In the first stage, some memory loss occurred, but the patient knew who and where he was. In the second stage, space and time were lost, but since the patient was aware that the change had occurred, there was much anxiety. In stage three, there was a loss of space and time and loss of all feeling that should be present. Cameron notes:

> During this stage the patient may show . . . loss of a second language or all knowledge of his marital status. . . . he may be unable to walk without support, to feed himself, and he may show double incontinence. . . . all schizophrenic symptomatology is absent. His communications are brief and rarely spontaneous, his replies to questions are in no way conditioned by recollections of the past or by anticipations of the future. He is completely free from all emotional disturbance save for a customary mild euphoria. He lives, as it were, in a very narrow segment of time and space.

Cameron would move the patients back and forth between these stages. In the only follow-up study that he carried out, the results clearly did not justify the means. Psychological follow-up testing demonstrated that schizophrenic thinking was still present although the patients did not necessarily demonstrate abnormal behavior. Cameron developed a theory to explain this fact, namely, that the brain has "surplus capacities" that take over. He suggested that the brain utilizes other processes to hide the abnormalities in thinking and the behaviors that result from disturbed perception. A warning is included, however, that this "new organization can be disturbed and, in particular, can be disturbed by emotional stress."

Cameron was quite adept at developing theories to explain

brain behavior, such as his concept of the "switcher device," which allowed individuals to ignore intrusive messages—an explanation he used to understand why his patients fought off the psychic driving tapes. Unfortunately, he was not capable of testing these hypotheses in any scientific manner, often because of his own biases. Thus he saw healthy coping mechanisms as stubborn attempts on the part of the patients to frustrate his objectives.

Another of his theories was the concept of the "contra-trait." He postulated that underlying every neurotic trait lay a more healthy contra-trait. Thus the contra-trait of passivity would be assertiveness. The goal of psychic driving was to activate these so-called contra-traits. Cameron and his colleagues explored all dimensions of this approach; they were able to demonstrate that the driving process could produce physiological responses observable by muscle measurement. There was concern, however, that any changes in attitude or emotional state were short-lived. By 1958, in an attempt to make these changes long-lasting, reinforcement procedures were developed so that the patient would listen to the verbal messages on a regular basis for weeks or months. They also decided that patients should be removed from the disturbed family environments that fostered the negative behavior, so that some patients were sent to foster homes for up to three months after discharge from the hospital.

From 1959 through 1962, attempts were made to simplify the procedure, to develop more valid methods of assessment, and to produce permanent change in those patients who underwent this treatment. Special attention was paid to the issues of how the patient should be prepared for driving, innovative approaches to the preparation of the verbal driving messages, and the ways in which exposure would be most effective. As previously noted, Cameron's early work focused on depatterning, with repeated electroshock and prolonged sleep as the principal methods used to break down the ongoing neurotic patterns and reduce the patient's "critical awareness." Cameron continued to feel that these were the most appropriate approaches in the most difficult cases. At this time, however, Cameron began to build on a method that had its origins in the psychology department of McGill University.

D. O. Hebb, one of the world's great psychologists, was chairman of the psychology department during these years. Hebb and his research group had a particular interest in the influence of sensory stimulation on animal development, in particular, mental development and the ability to learn. This interest gave rise to a series of experiments that were designed to examine how humans are dependent on their environment for the stimulation it provides—stimulation that, in turn, activates our mental processes. This led to the design of an experiment that ushered in the era of sensory deprivation research.

College student volunteers were paid $20 a day to spend time in a cubicle that was partially soundproofed. They lay on a bed with their eyes covered by a translucent plastic shield (allowing light by no patterned vision); hands were enclosed in tubes to prevent their being used for touch sensation; ears were covered with earphones from which there was a constant buzzing; a foam-rubber U-shaped cushion cradled the head and covered the ears. The students remained in this fashion except to eat or go to the bathroom. Most of the students could tolerate this procedure for only two or three days; the maximum was six.

The effects on these twenty-two male students were startling. Boredom gave way to restlessness and an inability to concentrate; problem solving was impaired; visual hallucinations and disturbances of body awareness began to occur; feelings of being detached from their bodies, or "depersonalization," developed. Hebb notes, "The subject's very identity had begun to disintegrate." Subsequent work showed that, while in this condition, students would listen to material that they would normally treat with contempt, such as information on the occult. Interest in such oddities persisted afterward in some of the subjects.

Further work in sensory deprivation was carried out, primarily in the United States. Interest was high because of concerns about the effects of space flight on astronauts, because of the effects on some patients of the monotonous experience of being in a respirator, and also because of the potential use of sensory deprivation in interrogation. The state of the art was summarized in a symposium held at Harvard University in 1958. George Ruff of the United States Air Force made a comment that, as we shall see, had significant implications for the work of Cameron: "Although no studies have yet been reported in which the subject is not allowed to leave the chamber if he 'wants out,' it seems likely that such an experiment would produce behavior unlike that observed where an escape route is available." It is striking that none of the research on sensory deprivation involved the use of patients. Subjects were volunteers and often screened for healthy emotional functioning prior to the experiments. It is also clear that nowhere was this procedure seen as a treatment for emotional disturbance.

In a May 1960 paper prepared for a United States Air Force conference on space flight and astronaut selection, Cameron described how the early work on isolation was utilized by his group at the Allan Memorial. Three series of experiments were conducted: the first involved the reduction of extrinsic stimuli through eyes, ears, and hands; the second, reduction of sensory input by interfering with the passage of stimuli from sensory receptors (the specialized nerve endings that receive messages from the outside world) to the brain; the third, reduction of the level of awareness of patients so as to make them less responsive to stimulation.

In the first series of experiments, the Allan group, led by Hassan Azima, used patients as experimental subjects in an attempt to understand their psychodynamic processes and to elicit underlying conflicts. To this end, patients were kept in sensory isolation for one to seven days. Cameron extended this period for up to sixteen days. (In his own files, there are reports of up to thirty-five days.) He noted similar responses to those described initially by Hebb on volunteers who were isolated for considerably less time.

Cameron realized that if patients were given a definite time period in isolation, they could tolerate the experience better than if no time-structuring was offered. In his papers is the following note:

> We should realize that our time structuring of sensory iso-

> lation is quite different from that of the Department of Psychology and all others since theirs was a self-imposed stay, whereas in ours, the length of stay is imposed from outside and that we have also got two categories, namely, that we have got one in which some structuring is given in terms of the staff saying "Oh well, it won't be much longer," or "It will be a week or so," or something of that kind, whereas with strict sensory isolation and *the staff being forced to say nothing* it was indefinite and therefore much more disturbing.

Ruff's comment concerning the absence of escape routes had proved prophetic.

The second series of experiments revolved around attempts to diminish the conduction of stimuli within the body. In this work, the experimental drug Sernyl (PCP) was used. The effects included apathy, anxiety, disturbed body image, unreality and depersonalization, thought disorder, disorganization, hallucinations, paranoia, and catatonia.

Third, in attempts to reduce further the activity of the patients, the depatterning experiments utilizing massive shock treatment were developed. Cameron also immobilized patients by injecting them with curare in beeswax, and even reported placing patients under heat lamps so that the warmth would increase receptivity.

So by 1961 Cameron was using sensory deprivation, prolonged sleep plus sensory deprivation, massive ECT plus sleep and various drugs such as PCP and curare to immobilize patients—all in order to facilitate their receptivity to driving statements. In notes made in March 1960 in preparation for the Texas conference on space flight, Cameron suggested some other factors that he thought would be worthy of investigation with respect to sensory deprivation. These included use of sensory overload, such as sound or light, pain, and verbal stimulation. There is no record of this work having been undertaken.

In conjunction with the work on sensory deprivation, Cameron and his group spent considerable time modifying the format in which the verbal signals were given. One of the members of the research group notes that every Wednesday Cameron would meet with his colleagues and they would review the cases and modify the techniques. They experimented with signals in which there were variation in voices (male and female), intervals, pauses, emphases, and changes in attitudes. In addition, they experimented with the alternation of self-destructive and supportive messages. The destructive messages, termed "negative driving," contained statements that rephrased the bad feelings that patients had expressed about themselves. For example, a typical series of statements might be, "You were a selfish husband. You only thought of your own needs. You were never around when the children needed you." Supportive messages, termed "positive driving," represented changes that either the patient or the therapist thought would improve the patient's life. Positive statements might include such phrases as "You are a warm, lovable person. People are attracted to you because of your humor. You reach out to others." The negative comments were played first for about ten days; as patients became increasingly hostile (explained as the activation of contra-traits), they were switched to positive comments. Cameron noted: "It is estimated that the negative and positive signals combined are repeated between one quarter and one half million times during the course of the exposure." The positive driving also lasted about ten days, and once again the patients became restless. This was explained as their wanting to be up and out, using their newly found patterns of response! He reported that they had kept the positive driving going for up to sixty or seventy days; there is in his notes a report of one woman who listened to the positive statements for one hundred and one consecutive days.

In 1964, in a paper published in *Comprehensive Psychiatry*, Cameron described a new technique in which the patients were no longer expected to be totally passive. They were now required to write down their thoughts at various times as the tapes played: "Writing out requires that the patient should think about the matter, should assemble his feeling and impressions in conceptual form and should express them in a manner aimed at the grasp and understanding of the reader." One woman later reported that she filled notebook after notebook with written material hoping to please Dr. Cameron.

On discharge from the hospital, patients would continue to listen to these tapes on a regular basis in order to reinforce the behavior change. Once again, Cameron's comment is revealing: "It begins to assume similarities to the other forms of meditation and self-criticism and evaluation such as is found in certain religions and in some political systems." This comment can only allude to the methods utilized by the Chinese Communists to effect attitude and behavior change in their compatriots following the takeover of the Mainland in 1949. It is also an allusion to what was then known about the techniques used to coerce American prisoners of war (POWs) into making false confessions during the Korean War. The parallels appear to be more than coincidence.

The assessment of change continued to be problematic. Most of the evaluation relied on the subjective responses of patients, staff, or family. Cameron himself called this a "fundamental weakness" of the experiments. Consequently, attempts were made to utilize such techniques as psychological tests and galvanic skin reflex tests (a standardized physiological test to measure responses to key words or phrases), sound movies made before and after driving, measurement of physiological responses such as heart rate, and electronic analyses of the vocal productions of the subjects. Although these assessments still did not conclusively demonstrate the efficacy of Cameron's methods, he persisted in seeing his work as revolutionizing treatment; it was, he said, "an alternative to the laborious, low efficiency methods . . . through ordinary psychotherapy."

Comments of Cameron's colleagues twenty years later suggest that many, even at the time, neither agreed with nor approved of his methods. During an interview, I was told by one of Cameron's colleagues that "a lot of people felt that it was a lot of crap—but we couldn't do anything." This man also noted that Cameron "didn't know the difference between good and poor research or treatment. . . . Dr. Cameron had the greatness of mediocrity with flashes of brilliance." One of Cameron's closest colleagues felt that the experiments were not properly set up and that the therapies were "things which were picked up from the circus." Another man who was very familiar with the work states that "there was a lot of opposition . . . but not to his face. . . . No one would speak out against Cameron." In a 1982 paper on the history of psychiatry at McGill, R. A. Cleghorn, Cameron's successor, commented: "It is apparent that Cameron's entrepreneurial skills, so successful in the organization of teaching and training, were not so appropriate in research." D. O. Hebb, during his last interview before his death in the summer of 1985, was not so kind:

> Cameron was irresponsible . . . criminally stupid. . . . There was no reason to expect that he would get any results. . . . He wanted to make a name for himself—so he threw his cap over the windmill. . . . It wasn't so much that he wanted to know—it was that he was driven with wanting to be important.

Depatterning and psychic driving was a treatment regimen that occupied Cameron from the early 1950s through 1962. It was based upon premises that had no physiological or psychological validity. Most striking, the hypotheses upon which these procedures were based were at marked variance to all that Cameron had written with respect both to memory and treatment at an earlier point in his career. In his monograph *Remembering*, published in 1947, he rejected the concept of the mind as a *tabula rasa* or as a storehouse of memories that can be brought out on demand or that can be mislaid or forgotten through carelessness. He emphasized that the key aspect both for the formation of a memory and for its recall is the frame of reference at the time of the event. In order for us to remember an experience or a face and to later recall that event or person, the mind must be sufficiently alert and focused so that the physiological processes that constitute the formation of memories can occur. He noted then that the use of ECT, insulin, sodium amytal, and other adjuvants (drugs that disinhibit) affects the ability to remember. He felt that amytal interviews were of limited usefulness because the

> remembering . . . is not accompanied by strong, emotional

> reactions. . . . [the thinking] is rarely accompanied by expansion of the topic and its integration with others and by subsequent rumination and reminiscences which are necessary to adequate remembering.

He went on to describe how full reactivity or responsiveness at the time is necessary for an individual to remember an event.

In therapy, the underlying premise is that much deviant behavior depends upon memory, and reactivation of the memories is necessary for behavior change to occur. This reactivation must take place when the individual is fully operative. Therefore, such drugs as sodium amytal are of limited usefulness in achieving permanent behavior change. Cameron, however, had other ideas. Over five years he attempted to produce behavior and attitudinal change on individuals whose brains were hardly capable of assimilating the messages of the tape recordings. The discrepancy between Cameron's lifelong work in memory and his diametrically opposed approach to treatment is one of the great mysteries of this man and his story.

In previous pages I have attempted to reconstruct the symptoms that my father displayed when he began recurring treatment at the Allan Memorial Institute. Given these problems, it is possible to develop a likely diagnosis. In addition, a survey of the textbooks of the time indicates the most reasonable approach to treatment that a patient with that diagnosis might have received in any reputable institution in the United States and Canada.

Diagnoses tend to be bound to the knowledge of emotional disturbance and the state of the psychiatric art at the time. In the 1950s, the most reasonable explanation for my father's symptoms would have been that of an anxiety neurosis—basically, the diagnosis that he was given. Such a disturbance consists of symptoms of generalized anxiety that are persistent over an extended period of time. The symptoms might include signs of muscular tension as manifested by restlessness, pacing, and a complete inability to relax. One would also see signs of physiological response to stress—a racing heart, sweating, rapid breathing, and similar disturbances. Such a patient might be afflicted with anxiety, excessive and nameless fears, inability to sleep, and problems in concentration. What are not part of this kind of picture are feelings of loss of reality, paranoia, hallucinations, or other bizarre symptoms of more serious disorders such as schizophrenia.

During the 1950s, an acute disorder such as I have described might have been treated with a combination of moderate sedation with a barbiturate in conjunction with an intensive attempt at psychotherapy. It is my opinion that the extreme physical procedures used on my father at the Allan represented a massive departure from the accepted psychodynamic methods for overcoming resistance and eliciting hidden thoughts and emotions. The escalation of procedures designed to break him down and demolish his defenses was such a departure from reasonable treatment that its use is incomprehensible. The continued assault on physiological functioning was simply unacceptable given the recent onset of symptoms and the diagnosis that he was given. A more judicious approach would have left him considerably better off, and likely in good health today.

If my father were to present his original symptoms to a psychiatrist today, I believe that the diagnosis might be different. At this time he might be diagnosed as experiencing a panic disorder. In current psychiatric parlance, such a disturbance is characterized by the occurrence of discrete episodes of panic that take place within a specified period of time. The precipitants of the panic are not clearly external, and a variety of symptoms might be included, such as shortness of breath, experience of choking, chest discomfort, skipped heart beats, and fear of dying. This diagnosis could not have been given in the 1950s, since our knowledge of the panic syndrome and the factors that contribute to its onset is relatively recent. Today's treatment might include the administration of medications such as antidepressants and a specific antianxiety drug, both of which seem to work on the disorder. Combining these with a psychotherapeutic approach that might incorporate principles of behavioral modification designed to overcome fears and teach ways of responding to the attacks would offer a reasonable hope that treatment would be successful. I would like to emphasize, however, that even with the dearth of knowledge and the small choice in available medications during the 1950s, the treatment given at the Allan was not only inappropriate but ultimately physically and emotionally destructive.

What kind of man would experiment on vulnerable patients? Ewen Cameron, it is said, came from a background where much was expected of him. His life became focused upon success and fame; he was determined to excel, and it is clear that the accolades of his colleagues were an important part of his motivation. He grew up as an authoritarian personality, a man who took delight in his power to make decisions that would greatly influence the lives of others, be they colleagues or patients. This need to be in control, when combined with a desire to succeed, could readily produce a situation in which he would make up his mind to conquer a disease that had baffled everyone—schizophrenia. He was so intolerant of weakness in others that the symptoms of patients goaded him to carry out procedures that would eliminate the offending behaviors. Missionary zeal rapidly slid into a process of dehumanizing the very patients that he was trying to save. How else can one explain his use of extreme measures on patients whose illnesses were far less severe than last-stage schizophrenia?

Toward the end of his life, he is said to have commented that he wished to "crack RNA" and to climb the mountain on which he ultimately died. Scaling new heights was the dominant force in his life—but he climbed that mountain on the backs of victims like my father.

9

Supply and Demand

I now had a fairly complete understanding of what Ewen Cameron was trying to do, and I even had some sense of what his motivations might have been. But there remained a piece of the puzzle yet to be fixed in place. How was it that a psychiatrist in Canada was chosen by the Central Intelligence Agency of the United States to receive money for research? Clearly, a commonality of interest had emerged; it was this relationship that I needed to explore.

The seeds of the relationship lie in the growth in intelligence work beginning in World War II. Much of this work has been well described elsewhere, but a brief history of the evolution of the American intelligence community will reveal the fertile ground that promoted the growth of mind-control experimentation.

In 1940, President Roosevelt sent William "Wild Bill" J. Donovan, a New York attorney and World War I general, on a fact-finding mission to Europe. The United States had not yet developed an intelligence-gathering capacity similar to that of many of the European nations. With the fast-moving events of World War II and the sudden involvement of the United States in the world arena, there was much to be learned, and quickly. Donovan returned with a proposal to establish a centralized intelligence unit to be called the Office of Coordinator of Information, with himself as director. It had two divisions: the Office of Strategic Services (OSS) and the Office of War Information. The OSS quickly developed relationships with members of the scientific community of the United States who offered their expertise in a variety of fields, from the use of chemical and biological substances to the use of hypnosis. Richard Helms, later to become director of the CIA, was an early recruit to this work.

In 1946, President Truman established the National Intelligence Authority (NIA), which was similar to the present-day National Security Council. Within this agency, a Central Intelligence Group was formed to oversee the gathering of data. Momentum increased, and in 1947 the Central Intelligence Agency (CIA) was established through the National Security Act. Truman was clearly ambivalent about the establishment of the CIA; as noted in Merle Miller's biography, he said: "Secrecy and a free, democratic government don't mix."

The history of officially sanctioned mind-control experimentation in the United States began in 1950, when the Director of Central Intelligence approved the establishment of a project, code-named Bluebird. Its objectives were as follows:

- To discover means of conditioning personnel to prevent unauthorized extraction of information from them by known means
- To investigate the possibility of control of an individual by application of special interrogation techniques
- To study memory enhancement
- To establish defensive means for preventing hostile control of Agency personnel.

Subsequently, a fifth objective was added:

- To evaluate offensive uses of unconventional interrogation techniques, including hypnosis and drugs

In 1951, the CIA decided to coordinate efforts with the U.S. Army, Navy, and Air Force, and Project Artichoke was born. A 1952 memorandum describes its mission as follows:

- Evaluation and development of any method by which we can get information from a person against his will and without his knowledge.
- How can we counter the above measures if they are used against us?
- Can we get control of an individual to the point where he will do our bidding against his will and even against such fundamental laws of nature such as self-preservation?
- How could we counter such measures if they are used against us?

Work was to include in-house experiments on interrogation techniques as well as interrogation of individuals overseas who had been apprehended by the CIA. The idea was to utilize these newer techniques such as drugs and hypnosis to facilitate the extracting of information from foreign nationals. A remarkably wide variety of substances were examined, including narcotics, mushrooms, truth sera, cocaine, amphetamines, barbiturates, nitrous oxide, and many others.

In 1953, Project Artichoke evolved into Project MKULTRA, the major CIA program of research on substances designed to influence behavior, a program that was to last for almost twenty years. Richard Helms has been described as the driving force behind this endeavor, and in a 1953 memo he noted that part of its function was "implanting suggestions and other forms of mental control." MKULTRA was to move from laboratory testing on animals to testing on human volunteers (although the individuals were not necessarily to know what substance they were ingesting) and to the use of experimental drugs on totally unknowing citizens. The range of experiments that the CIA developed to test these materials is both horrifying and fascinating. At least one death can be attributed to the work; more may have occurred. Many lives were touched, and some subjects live on with the effects of MKULTRA disturbing their ability to think.

All this remained hidden from the general public until Tuesday, August 2, 1977, when the *New York Times* published a front page article with the headline "Private Institutions Used In CIA Effort To Control Behavior." I still find it difficult to believe that I heard nothing about this report until two years later, when I came across the review of John Marks's book. In the midst of a job change, my attentions were obviously elsewhere.

The *Times* piece described a secret twenty-five year and twenty-five million dollar project—MKULTRA—designed to investigate methods to influence memory, thought, attitude, motivation, and ultimately human behavior. Several prominent psychiatrists were associated with this project—one of them was Ewen Cameron. The article described CIA and U.S. armed services attempts at new methods of interrogation and brainwashing, and revealed that CIA money had been laundered through at least three funding conduits: the Society for the Investigation of Human Ecology, founded at Cornell University; the Geschicter Foundation for Medical Research; and the Josiah Macy Foundation. Cameron's work was labeled brainwashing, and an interview with Leonard Rubenstein, Cameron's assistant, was included. Rubenstein noted: "They had investigated brainwashing among soldiers who had been in Korea. We in Montreal started to use some [of these] techniques, brainwashing patients instead of [using] drugs." He went on to describe experiments in sensory deprivation.

On the day following the public revelations, Admiral Stansfield Turner, then Director of Central Intelligence, was called to testify before a joint hearing of the Select Committee on Intelligence and the Subcommittee on Health and Scientific Research of the Committee on Human Resources of the United States Senate. For the first time, he revealed the contents of several thousand documents related to mind-control research that had recently been discovered in response to a Freedom of Information request by the author John Marks. The statistics were impressive: 185 nongovernment researchers in eighty institutions were involved. Forty-four colleges and universities, fifteen research foundations, twelve hospitals and clinics, and three penal institutions served as the sites where this work had been carried out. The projects were wide-ranging but were bound together by a common goal—the need to influence and gain control over memory and human behavior. The projects included the following:

- Research into the effects of behavioral drugs and/or alcohol
- Research on hypnosis
- Acquisition of chemicals or drugs
- Aspects of magicians' art useful in covert operations, for example, surreptitious delivery of drug-related material
- Studies of human behavior, sleep research, and behavioral changes during psychotherapy
- Polygraph research
- Research on toxins, drugs, and biologicals in human tissues; provision of exotic pathogens and the capability to incorporate them in effective delivery systems (in other words, germ warfare)
- Effects of shock treatment, harassment techniques for offensive use, and gas-propelled sprays and aerosols
- Chemical and biological warfare techniques involving the army

Examples were included in Turner's description of the projects. He noted that many of these experiments were carried out on human subjects—some of whom were volunteers, many of whom were not.

Enter Ewen Cameron. The origins of his association with MKULTRA can be traced early enough. Experimentation requires funding. Although Cameron's patients paid for their "treatment," their money was, of course, channeled to the hospital. Consequently, outside funding sources were a necessity for the work to continue. It is here that the tangled relationship between the Cold War of the 1950s and the work of Ewen Cameron becomes clear; the old adage "politics makes strange bedfellows" aptly describes this case. Cameron's first paper on psychic driving appeared in the *American Journal of Psychiatry* in 1956; its principal message was that behavior could be affected by exposure to repetition of taped messages—and it brought him to the attention of the CIA. Why was the CIA so interested in this paper?

The answer lies in the subject of brainwashing, a term that was coined by a journalist, Edward Hunter, in an article that appeared in the *Miami Daily News* in 1950. Hunter's use of the term and his writings about its use in China blended well with the Cold War fears of Chinese and Russian abilities to influence attitude and behavior. Hunter was an anticommunist who worked covertly for the CIA. His book, *Brainwashing in Red China*, served to fan the flames of anticommunist hysteria and thereby allowed the CIA and the U.S. armed services to embark on a twenty-year project designed to develop indoctrination techniques.

American interest in interrogation had begun during the Soviet "show trials" of the 1930s when stalwart party members publicly declared themselves to be traitors. In 1949 Cardinal Mindszenty's trial in Hungary revealed a man broken by some untoward experience, mouthing words that were entirely foreign to the person he was known to be. A later event—one that was to be of great consequence to the CIA—provided further impetus to brainwashing research. The American ambassador to the Soviet Union, George Kennan, came to Berlin from Moscow and, as Richard Helms describes it, made a series of extraordinary statements that were regarded by the people in the State Department as quite uncharacteristic. They suspected that he had been given something—possibly a drug—by the Russians.

The concern about brainwashing reached its peak during the Korean War. Not only were the Chinese reported to be able to obtain signed confessions from American prisoners of war, but American pilots made seemingly uncoerced radio broadcasts accepting guilt for their war activities. Whether these examples actually took place is not entirely clear. What did happen is that brainwashing was sensationalized in the American media and used to heighten the American public's anticommunist feeling. It became a rationalization for chemical and psychological research into interrogation techniques.

As these concerns heated up, a working group was set up by the Air Force under the leadership of a man named Fred Williams. This group, the Air Force Psychological Warfare Division, was located at Maxwell Air Force Base in Montgomery, Alabama, and was part of a network attempting to understand the implications of the POW confessions. Among those associated with this group, several ultimately became involved in mind control research, including Colonel James Monroe (who was later to join the CIA); Albert Biderman, a sociologist; Harold Wolff and Lawrence Hinkle at Cornell; and CIA psychologist John Gittinger. Wolff was a nationally known neurologist who had made the acquaintance of Allen Dulles, director of the CIA, when he treated Dulles's son for injuries suffered during the Korean war. It was Wolff and Hinkle who produced the major treatise on brainwashing that emerged during this period. Originally written as a report for the Technical Services Division of the CIA in 1956, it was published in a major psychiatric journal, the *Archives of Neurology and Psychiatry*, in the same year under the title "Communist Interrogation and Indoctrination of 'Enemies of the State': Analysis of Methods Used by the Communist State Police (A Special Report)."

The major contribution of this work lay in the revelation that it was not drugs or bizarre tortures that resulted in confession; the procedures rather made use of psychological knowledge and techniques that produced anxiety to such a degree that normal coping devices could not prevail. The role of the interrogator as friend and savior grew out of the need on the part of the prisoner to escape from the disintegration of his personality. Solitary confinement, sleep deprivation, and lack of information combined with skillful interrogation produced the desired outcome in almost every case. The Russians had initially developed this approach, and the Chinese had modified it by adding the element of group pressure. Conformity to a peer group's attitudes was of course part of the Chinese plan to convert its populace after they had taken control of mainland China. This technique was ultimately to prove eminently successful with the American POWs.

Although Wolff and Hinkle documented a process that was based on psychological understanding of the personality and group dynamics, they nevertheless concluded that there was "no evidence that psychologists, neurophysiologists, or other scientists participated in their development." Their revelations did, however, inspire the military and intelligence services to begin to formulate their own plans for the study of mind control. In 1954, Project QK-Hilltop was begun at Cornell Medical College under the direction of Harold Wolff—a spinoff from Monroe's group at Maxwell. Wolff had major interests in the area of stress, as well as in the interrelationships of man and his environment, a discipline that he called "human ecology." This approach, which integrated the interests of both behavioral and social scientists, could be used, he thought, not only to understand human behavior but ultimately to influence it. Proposing to examine every known method of influence and control, he asked that the CIA provide him with all its information on interrogation and intimidation:

> . . . including threats, coercion, imprisonment, deprivation, humiliation, torture, "brainwashing," "black psychiatry," hypnosis and combinations of these, with or without chemical agents. We will assemble, collate, analyze and assimilate this information and will then undertake experimental investigations designed to develop new techniques of offensive/defensive intelligence use. . . . Potentially useful secret drugs (and various brain damaging procedures) will be similarly tested in order to ascertain the fundamental effect upon human brain function and upon the subject's mood. . . . Where any of the studies involve potential harm to the subject, we expect the Agency to make available suitable subjects and a proper place for the performance of necessary experiments.

In other words, Wolff was not willing to expose his patients to harmful materials, but was willing to test them on other "suitable subjects."

In 1955 the CIA study group became the Society for the Investigation of Human Ecology based at Cornell, and was destined to serve as a major funding conduit from the CIA to behavioral science researchers across the United States, Canada, and Europe. The work that was undertaken has been well described in Marks's book *The Search for the Manchurian Candidate*. In 1957 the Society severed its ties with Cornell, although Hinkle and Wolff remained on its board. Colonel James Monroe became executive secretary of the organization as the CIA took an even greater role in its functioning. Sidney Gottlieb, the man most responsible for MKULTRA and one of its major funding arms, the Society, states:

> The Society would try to keep in touch with that part of the scientific research community which were in areas that we were interested in—usually its mode was to find somebody that was working in an area in which we were interested and encourage him to continue in that area with some funding from us.

Even prior to the formation of the Society, the American intelligence services had been interested in work done at McGill. Donald Hebb was chairman of the Human Relations and Research Committee of the Canadian Defence Research Board in 1950–51. As such, he was invited to attend a meeting of representatives of the British, Canadian, and American governments who at that time were concerned about the ability of the Soviet Union to elicit confessions from its own citizens. They conjectured that the Soviets were using some new psychological techniques. Shortly thereafter, Hebb began to wonder about the use of sensory deprivation as a tool for breaking people down. He subsequently received about $10,000 a year from the Canadian Defence Research Board to develop his work on sensory deprivation. Carried on by Hebb's students, the results were, as previously noted, quite startling: volunteer students placed in sensory isolation for over two to three days became depersonalized and unable to think, and they experienced hallucinations; they were then receptive to attitudinal change.

The work somehow came to the attention of members of the Canadian Parliament, who heard only that government money was being paid to students to lie around. Since the results had been classified, the work was quickly dropped. Hebb stated in an interview that the Defence Research Board stopped the funding either because of a loss of interest or because of a fear that it could be "trouble-making." Hebb also said in that interview that information on the work was "snatched immediately to some organization in the States."

Although Hebb himself felt that the work was boring and moved quickly on to other areas of intellectual pursuit, there continued to be great interest in the subject of sensory deprivation—both in the United States and in Canada.

John Gittinger, the CIA psychologist who was a staff member of the Society, saw Ewen Cameron's article on psychic driving and suggested to James Monroe that he contact Cameron. That same year Maitland Baldwin, a CIA-funded researcher in sensory deprivation, visited Cameron in Montreal "to discuss isolation techniques," and three months later a grant application was received by the Society from the Allan Memorial Institute.

The application was entitled "The Effects Upon Human Behavior of the Repetition of Verbal Signals." In it Cameron describes the procedures that he had developed at the Allan Memorial Institute:

> 1. The breaking down of ongoing patterns of the patient's behavior by means of particularly intensive electroshocks (depatterning).
> 2. The intensive repetition (16 hours a day for 6–7 days) of the prearranged verbal signal.
> 3. During this period of intensive repetition the patient is kept in partial sensory isolation.
> 4. Repression of the driving period is carried out by putting the patient, after the conclusion of the period, into continuous sleep for 7–10 days.

He then went on to describe the objectives of the proposal to the Society. The proposed study would find and test chemical agents that would serve "to break down ongoing patterns of behaviour more rapidly, more transitorily, and with less damage to the cognitive and perceptive capacities" of the patients. He would improve the recording mechanisms by using such techniques as multiple voices so as "to capitalize on the force of group decision and suggestion"; he planned to deactivate the patients and yet keep them at a higher activity level during driving by using such drugs as Artane, curare, Anectine, bulbocapnine, LSD 25, and similar experimental agents. These were seen as potentially more effective than electroshock and sleep.

In 1977 Gittinger, testifying before the joint hearing of the Select Committee on Intelligence and the Subcommittee on Health and Scientific Research of the Committee on Human Resources of the United States Senate, stated:

> By 1962 and 1963, the general idea we were able to come up with is that brainwashing was largely a process of isolating a human being, keeping him out of contact, putting him out of control, putting him under long stress in relationship to interviewing and interrogation, and that they could produce any change that way without having to resort to any kind of esoteric means.

If Cameron's work is examined with this formulation in mind, we see some startling parallels both to the brainwashing techniques described by Hinkle and Wolff, and to Gittinger's description. In Cameron's system, patients were subjected to long periods of sensory isolation, staff was not permitted to tell them for how long they would be there, staff asked the patients on a regular basis to repeat what they had heard, and patients were told to write down on a periodic basis all the thoughts associated with the verbal repetitions. As a result of either physical, chemical, or psychological treatments, patients were left confused, vulnerable, and open to hearing repeated messages. Several voices would be heard at once, simulating the pressure of a group. Cameron's work therefore appears to have been built on knowledge generated from research on brainwashing and sensory deprivation.

Albert Biderman, the CIA and Air Force sociologist, described the techniques of "Communist Coercive Methods for Eliciting Individual Compliance" in a 1957 article in the *Bulletin of the New York Academy of Medicine*; a similar report appeared in a paper prepared for the United States Air Force entitled "Communist Techniques of Coercive Interrogation." Biderman described eight general methods of coercion used on American POWs, their effects and their variations. The methods—which bear a striking resemblance to Cameron's techniques—were:

- *Isolation:* According to Biderman, the POW was removed

from his group and kept by himself. My father was placed in a darkened and quiet room by himself in a special part of the hospital.

- *Monopolization of perception:* Biderman was here making reference to a process of cutting off stimulation from the environment. POWs were kept in physical isolation with restricted movement, monotonous food, and darkness. My father was placed in a condition of partial sensory deprivation, which also results in markedly reduced perception of surroundings and a focusing of attention upon the internal processes of thinking and body sensations.
- *Induced debilitation or exhaustion:* Illness was induced in the POW by procedures designed to produce exhaustion, such as prolonged interrogation or forcing him to write down all his thoughts. My father was made ill with shock treatments, drugs, and sleep. In addition, my father and other Cameron patients were told to fill notebooks with their thoughts as they listened to voices. The patients were forced to listen to the recorded messages sixteen hours a day—loud voices, soft, male, female, multiples of voices pressuring patients who had been rendered confused and defenseless.
- *Threats* were another element of the brainwashing process. POWs were exposed to all kinds of threats to themselves or their families. My father faced the threat of endless isolation with the possibility of being cut off from his family forever.
- *Occasional indulgences* or favors were offered to soften up the POWs. These might include special foods or exercise. My father was permitted rare telephone calls to our family or an occasional bath.
- *Demonstrating "omnipotence" and "omniscience":* The captors had complete control over the fate of the POWs; they had complete knowledge of their activities. My father waited anxiously for Cameron, since he had rendered the patients so totally dependent upon him. Cameron and his associates also demonstrated their complete control by having nurses question patients every two hours about what they were hearing on the psychic driving tapes.

- *Degradation* reinforced the helplessness of the POWs: they were not permitted to attend to personal hygiene, they were not allowed privacy, and they were subjected to insults and taunts. My father, like other Cameron patients, was made incontinent in bladder and bowel. At times he was fed through a tube. The patients endured insults through the psychic driving messages ("You're a bad mother"). Doctors and nurse entered their rooms at will; and my father's questions of them were ignored: "What do you want?" he would ask in vain. Powerlessness was magnified by this complete disregard for human dignity.
- *Enforcing trivial demands:* POWs were forced to obey detailed rules that governed even the simplest part of their days. My father and the other patients were forced to remain in their cubicles, go to the toilet on demand, eat when told to, and obey Cameron's instructions without question.

Although I could clearly see the parallels between the reports of Chinese Communist brainwashing procedures and Cameron's work, I was still unable to make a tight connection between the two. Cameron had made allusions in his papers to these reports, but such evidence was not sufficient. Once again, in 1986, I returned to the archives of the American Psychiatric Association, which had the only papers of Ewen Cameron that were available to me. I was determined to find some clue.

It was my last morning in Washington. I had one hour to look again. Wearily, I took down the boxes of materials and began once more to review their contents. I idly picked up a rather obscure paper titled "The Transition Neurosis," a paper that Cameron had given at the Fifth Annual Neuropsychiatric meeting in North Little Rock, Arkansas, in February 1953. As I leafed through the pages, my eyes caught one paragraph; my heart began to race as I read it more closely. This was it!

In the paper, Cameron discusses the theory that people can respond to any given stimulus with many patterns of response; he notes that usually one pattern dominates while the others become unconscious. He goes on:

> We may suspect that in the extraordinary political conversions which we have seen, particularly in the iron curtain countries, advantage is being taken of this fact to bring into prominence alternative patternings of behavior actually carried by the individual but never previously suspected by him or others as being present. The stress required to bring this about, at least as far as the political conversions are concerned, is capable of being developed only behind the iron curtain. Sargent (1951) has described what little we know of the dynamics of these political and religious conversions and has attempted to duplicate them, but from what we gather, with somewhat limited success. He used depleting emetics. *We have explored this procedure in one case, using sleeplessness, disinhibiting agents, and hypnosis.*

There it was in black and white. I was filled with excitement. I needed to obtain a copy of this page; I reached into my pocket but I had no change. The archivist had no change. My plane was due to leave. I became excited, anxious, worried. The archivist waved me off with a free copy of the document. I began to run down the street with the page in my hand, back to the lawyers' office. "I have the proof," I thought. I was so excited that I almost knocked over a woman as I crossed the road. I could see the headlines: "Mad psychiatrist attacks innocent woman on sidewalk." I tried to slow down but could barely contain myself. I reached the lawyers' building and found the office closed. But I knew where to find them—in the restaurant downstairs. And so I rushed in, making a grand entrance as I waved my page.

"He had tried it!" I shouted. "Here it is—on paper!"

When I returned home to California, I followed up Cameron's allusion to the work of William Sargent. In his book, *Battle for the Mind: A Physiology of Conversion and Brainwashing*, Sargent describes the processes by which religious conversion may occur:

> By increasing or prolonging stresses in various ways, or inducing physical debilitation, a more thorough alteration of the person's thinking processes may be achieved. . . . If the stress or the physical debilitation, or both, are carried one stage further, it may happen that patterns of thought and

> behavior, especially those of recent acquisition, become disrupted. New patterns can then be substituted, or suppressed patterns allowed to reassert themselves; or the subject may begin to think or act in ways that precisely contradict his former ones.

More specifically with respect to brainwashing, he notes:

> If a complete sudden collapse can be produced by prolonging or intensifying emotional stress, the cortical slate may be wiped clean temporarily of its more recently implanted patterns of behavior, perhaps allowing others to be substituted more easily.

The parallel with Cameron's theory of differential amnesia is striking, and the relationship to brainwashing is abundantly clear.

So by 1953 Cameron had begun to try his hand at brainwashing; the process that he had tentatively started in the early 1950s was to blossom into a wholesale attempt to erase minds and reprogram them. With the assistance of the CIA through its MKULTRA project, Cameron's assault on the personality developed unchecked by any ethical or moral concerns. Under the guise of treatment, innocent patients became victims of brainwashing research.

Why did Cameron commit himself to this work? If one considers the impact of the Nuremberg trials on him, some clues emerge. It appears that in the late 1940s and early 1950s, he became obsessed with a need to control social deviance and to prevent the transmission of negative traits and attitudes from parents to children. Did his later attempts to change human behavior represent his response to this concern? Cameron's presidential address to the American Psychiatric Association in 1953 suggests his involvement in the Cold War and his concerns about communism. Although he also used the opportunity to express his concerns about McCarthyism, Cameron held to a now familiar position—our best hope for a new world order and without hysteria, one without the totalitarianism of either the right or left, lies in science. With behavioral scientists as leaders, order would emerge from chaos. Were these attitudes a factor in his determination to change behavior? It seems likely.

The CIA had a ready ally in Ewen Cameron. With the aid of an American working in Canada, caught up in Cold War concerns, wanting to change society and with tremendous power and access to an almost unlimited supply of subjects, the CIA funded brainwashing experiments from 1957 to 1960.

The work continued until 1963. At least one hundred patients went through brainwashing procedures, obediently following the prescriptions of Canada's "most eminent" psychiatrist. In 1967, three years after Cameron's departure from the Allan Memorial Institute, a study by Alex Schwartzman and Paul Termansen was published by the Institute. This paper reviewed the results of the depatterning program and was commissioned by Cleghorn, Cameron's immediate successor. It looked at seventy-nine patients who had been hospitalized from 1956–63 and who had reached the third stage of depatterning. The findings were both interesting and troubling. Of these patients, 24% relapsed following depatterning while still in the hospital; physical complications ranging from "mild" to "severe" were associated with treatment in 23% of the cases; there were severe complications in 6%.

Most important, these researchers found that a pattern of frequent electroshock treatment during hospitalization was associated with poor clinical outcome, and the shorter the interval between the ECTs, the greater was the current memory impairment on a standardized test of measurement, the Wechsler Memory Scale. Of the twenty-seven patients tested on memory function, 63% depended on others for recall of past events. There was persisting amnesia for periods ranging from six months to ten years in 60% of these people. And so, the final study indicated permanent brain damage in a high proportion of these patients.

Why had this study not been done earlier? How had almost ten years of ever-increasing and intrusive experimentation gone by with no one intervening? Given Cameron's published concerns, was this, ironically, just a recapitulation of what had happened in Nazi Germany—a man with great power is not stopped by his underlings? Or did his colleagues simply not know what was taking place? The experiment ended, but for the victims and those who loved them, the pain continues.

The final word is from Sidney Gottlieb, under whom the MKULTRA project flourished. When asked why he had suggested to Richard Helms that the papers relating to MKULTRA and mind control research be destroyed, he commented: "It was clear to me, and I have been deposed on this before, that the project, the project MKULTRA[,] had not yielded any results of real positive value to the Agency. . . ."

10

Stitching the Pieces Together

By 1985–86, I felt as though I was living life on at least two levels—my daily life, and my life as it was in the 1950s. Each source of information was gathered into a square of brightly colored cloth: blues of depression, reds of passion, white of honor, and black of decay. I would have to sew these pieces together into a quilt of coherent understanding—for me, for my family, for all of us. Perhaps I could help to ensure that such a perversion of medical care would never occur again.

I began to consider, in a somewhat more dispassionate manner, what my relationship with my father had been and what it now consisted of. This man around whom my life had been built was a figure who provoked great ambivalence in me. I needed to accept his limitations and honor him for who he was. How could I overcome my anger toward him? With my patients it was easy to say, "You cannot change what was. Let it go. Accept and form a relationship with what is. If the anger destroys you, it is because you hold on to it." Perhaps it was so difficult because of the helplessness that pervaded our loss; we seemed to have no control as we saw my father slipping away. Of course, that is true of many illnesses; it is true of death. But in this situation, there was no adequate explanation, not for twenty-five years. Helplessness breeds anger and often that rage is misdirected. For years I went through life blaming my father; resentment colored our relationship until 1979. And then—truth. Did it bring relief? Could it change a twenty-year pattern of anger? No—and now that I realized what had transpired I was left with guilt for not having been more accepting, more understanding. Sometimes I wonder if, for my own sake, it would have been better if the truth had never been aired. I would have blithely continued to the end, secure in my resentment, justified in my need to keep my father far away. Now I must forge ties anew, finding whatever is left of my father as his life draws to a close.

He seems small and a little frail as I spy him coming up the ramp from the airplane. With his ample belly, trench coat, and stylish hat, he marches with a jaunty air. We kiss awkwardly.

"How was your trip? Was the flight smooth?" I ask.

"Wonderful," he exclaims, "Couldn't be better. The food was beautiful. I had my drink and read the paper. Who could ask for more?"

With a conspiratorial air, he whispers in my ear. "The woman beside me wouldn't stop talking. I think it was her first flight. I told her all about my son and daughter-in-law in San Francisco—how proud I am of them."

We walk to the baggage claim area. I am happy to see him but I am anticipating the tension that will arise as the old feelings return. We talk about the weather in Montreal and the weather in California. My sisters are well, as are their children. He is still experiencing the pains in his legs and has seen the doctor twice in the last month.

I drive quietly, reminding myself that he is now eighty years old. By the time we arrive at the house, I have heard about his diet, pains, bowel habits, and indigestion several times over. When we enter, my sons come forward to greet him. He kisses them perfunctorily as he greets Rhona.

"I feel great to be here with you children. Can I have some tea?" He then begins to tell Rhona many of the same stories that I have heard for the past forty minutes. This could be the egocentric preoccupation of an elderly man, I think, but no, it is more. This has been his conversation for thirty years. When I am with him, I long to be close, to hug him and tell him how much I love him, how sorry I am that his life turned out the way that it did. Sometimes, when he is unaware of my gaze, I watch him and my eyes fill up. He sits in the sun, smoking the omnipresent cigar, looking at the orange trees and flowers. In the twilight of his life, a shadow of the man I remember, he seems content.

But I remember; flashbacks to a man of stature, of confidence, a man whose jaunty walk was a reflection of a personality that radiated security. Images of me, a small ten-year-old walking quickly to catch up to him on the streets of New York. Our family is there for the Easter holiday, ensconced in a three-room suite at the Park Sheraton Hotel. My oldest sister, Frances, and her husband, Dan, are in a room next door. My father has taken us all to the big city. I look out the window at the tall buildings, the people down below. New York is strange and frightening to me, but for my father, New York is his kind of town—fast people, good times, music, clubs, excitement. My mother takes us to Radio City Music Hall; my father takes us to the El Morocco to hear my sister's favorite singer, Johnny Ray. She swoons; I laugh; my father jokes; my mother smiles. The air sparkles with electricity as we walk up Broadway. There are smoke rings coming out of that billboard; look at the waterfall! Times Square, people; life is discovery, and Daddy leads me to the challenge.

He still likes to go out to dinner. Rhona and I take him to a very special restaurant in San Francisco. We have to choose carefully because he will eat only a few things. Meat must be very tender, food very hot, and a cup of hot water must accompany his meal. With a sigh of relief, Rhona and I look at each other as we realize that he is enjoying his food. When we go for a walk and discuss the past, he tells me of the good times long ago. He recalls when the waiters in the best places knew him by name; he remembers the good times in New York. With a choking sob, he remembers my mother.

Sometimes I take his hand, and I feel the simultaneous explosion of love and anger. My emotions become tossed in a sea of boiling currents, whipped up by the winds of what might have been. I draw close; I retreat. I want so much for him to be at peace and yet, at other times, I turn on him suddenly with an anger so intense that its depth shocks even me. I try so hard to be a good son, and he sees me that way. I want my sons to see that respect and honor are the prerogative of age. Inside, it is as it has always been—I hide, recoiling in pain with a hunger that will never be satisfied.

Each year he visits for two weeks, grateful to escape the cold of a Montreal winter. Now, as part of my search for truth, I ask him more about the past.

Who were you before you met Cameron? Tell me more about how you and Mom met. Why did you name your business Teresa Frocks? Did you like your father? What was it like when they kept you asleep?

During one of these visits, he told me for the first time that he still hears the voice that he heard for days at the Allan Memorial Institute—endless repetitions that enter his consciousness as he lies in that twilight state between sleep and waking.

He does not know how much work I have done in trying to piece his story together. He is unaware of the many telephone calls and trips to Washington; the numerous letters, interviews; the work on the book. He is oblivious and I do not want him to know.

As I become more involved in the research concerning the CIA, Rhona begins to worry that I might bring to light things that I would be better off leaving in the darkness. I try to reassure her, but at one point she becomes convinced that our telephone is tapped. I feel that this is ridiculous, but given all that I have read about intelligence services here and abroad, I must agree that anything is possible. At one point I hear that the CIA attorney has asked about my book—*how do they know*? An air of paranoia begins to surround our house. I ask the lawyers in Washington if this is silly—they do not reassure me. We do not change our daily lives, but we become increasingly wary. For some months, my father has refused to talk with me on the telephone about the lawsuit against the CIA for fear that we are listened to. I attribute his concerns to his usual suspicion; now I am walking around with the same ideas. When I leave the country, I am certain that, at the moment of reentry, the immigration officer will tap into his computer, and say: "No, sir. I'm sorry. You are no longer welcome in the United States." For the first time in my life, I have a real sense of what the life of a paranoid person must be. Suddenly, one becomes the center of a world where the unknown is hostile, where danger lurks. The only difference between me and those whose lives are destroyed by their fears is that I know that this is all a manifestation of my preoccupation.

There is a fine line at times between those of us whose minds are clear and those whose reality is distorted by internal pain, rage, or terror. For many years I was haunted by a nightmare in which I was destined for the same end as my father. I too would reach my late forties and depression or anxiety or some other dread mental decay would set in; I would then retreat to some nether world of self-absorption where no one could enter. The first time the thought entered my mind was when I was fourteen; through my twenties and thirties, it was repressed. Then, shortly after my fortieth birthday, I became quite ill with a severe flu. Rhona was away in the East at a meeting and I was alone with the children. After I had sent them off to school, I returned to bed, feverish and having significant trouble breathing. As I lay there gasping for breath, I realized in terror that my hand was clutching at my breast.

"No!" I shouted, "Never."

The nightmare returned and became a part of my life once more.

It is an odd coincidence, but only recently has Rhona revealed to me that after my fortieth birthday, she, too, had developed the fear that my life would end as had my father's. I did not share my fantasy, not wanting to frighten her; she had held her fears close, not wanting to worry me. Today, we both feel that the transition to my forties, the decade in which my father's life was ruined, precipitated a resurgence of feelings and memories of my lost adolescence. Only as I overcame the helplessness of the past by involving myself in fighting the CIA in a court battle, as the paralysis of doing nothing turned into an active search for understanding, could I let the fear go.

How much of my father do I hold within me? Sometimes I find myself teasing my sons. The words that I use seem vaguely familiar; the jokes evoke scenes of other times, other places; the tone is not my own. I call my son "Bear"; my Dad would tease me when I needed a haircut by calling me "Bear." I sing with my boys—the melodies are the nonsense tunes that peppered my father's playful interaction with his children:

> I found a peanut
> Where did you find it?
> Right over there.
> What did it taste like?
> Just like a peanut!

He is within me, and yet we differ in a thousand ways. I do not search for security in material possessions; my joy lies in books or music, in a long hike or skiing over the hushed snow of a Sierra valley. My peace lies in the faces of my sons as I rehearse their lines with them for a school play. Not for me the card games, the night life, or the liquor; I search for stimulation in new places far away from the familiar. Our paths cross in the value we both place on family and friends; we diverge politically. I am of the first North American-born generation and I return to the religious values that he cast aside. So much the same, yet needing so much to be different, I am my father and mother; I am myself; I am father to my children. Generation to generation; we hold on; we let go; we remember; we forget. We accept.

My patient is a first-year graduate student at Stanford. At twenty-two, he looks no more than sixteen. His background is familiar, only New York Jewish instead of Montreal. He, too, lost a father, only to divorce instead of to Ewen Cameron. Anger and longing play across his face as he remembers.

"I hate him. How could he walk out? I tried to stop him. I held on to his coat on the stairs. Please, I cried, stay for me. Why do you have to go? I love you, Daddy, Don't go, don't. . . ."

He squirms in his chair; his fists are clenched as the shadows darken his mind. Tears appear at the corners of his eyes.

"I felt as though my world had ended. I ran to my room and began to break things. No one stopped me. Mom was in her room, filled with her own grief. I saw a photograph of him and me fishing. I lunged at it and threw it across the room at the wall. Never have I felt such pain. And no one stopped me, no one loved me; no one hugged me."

He is crying bitterly. As I sit in my chair, I feel as though I need to send out waves of comfort. Rooted in professional reserve, I make a comment that soothes and questions. I conjure up a mental image of a little boy, angry and afraid, and I go to him with warmth and concern. I pick up the child. His tense body relaxes as he lets go his tears. In my chair, I ask another question; in my mind, I tell the little boy a story. Multiple levels of conversation woven through layers of memory—the conscious, the preconscious, the unconscious—his, mine, ours.

In 1985–86, the past colored the present. At home, in my office, with family, friends, and patients, the quest became the core of my being. I became impatient in many social situations as my thoughts strayed elsewhere. I had little patience with the niceties of daily life; my feelings were too intense for the fine art of delicate conversation. Yet no one knew what I experienced every day. I had perfected my act a long time ago.

I began to realize that I needed to talk to others whose lives had been touched by Ewen Cameron. Perhaps I wanted to see if my father was unique; maybe I was looking for others who could understand my grief because of their own pain. It was time to leave my study and come face to face with the reality that lay outside my family. In the summer of 1986, I set off to interview some of the others whose lives had been irrevocably changed.

11

The Story of Jeanine Huard: Opportunities Lost

> I'm a dreamer. I always will be. I hope one day to be better; to do all the things I'd like to do. . . . I'd like to travel.

As I drove out of Montreal, I found it difficult to concentrate on the road. At times, my mind conjured up images of long ago—my mother taking care of me when I was ill; my father playing golf. I wondered what I was going to find when I arrived at my destination. My palms were sweaty on the wheel and I could not seem to find a comfortable place in the seat of the rental car. When I had first written from California, Jeanine Huard's response had taken a long time to arrive. When it did, the handwritten letter conveyed emptiness, apathy, and significant depression:

> My state of health has been deteriorating and of course everything that brings me back these horrors are a cause of

> stress and shock to me; also [the experience with] the journalists to whom I have given and still give interviews is very painful. I do it because I want justice to be done for my sufferings. I hope that this day is soon because the fight is very ill-making.

I called her the week prior to my visit to Montreal, but she continued to be hesitant about seeing me. In the interim, both she and my father had made depositions to the CIA in Montreal; having met my father, she was now slightly more willing to talk with me. After further telephone calls she agreed, and I set out at once to drive to the suburb where she lived, some distance from downtown Montreal.

This was going to be the first time that I would meet another of the nine plaintiffs engaged with my father in the lawsuit against the CIA. This would also be the first occasion on which I would talk with another of Cameron's patients. I must acknowledge that I was afraid; I truly did not want to hear about any more pain. Yet it was critical, if I wanted to have a better understanding of what had transpired, to talk with patients as well as Cameron's colleagues.

When I reached her town, I stopped for some coffee and examined the map. I'm not a journalist, I thought, what am I doing here? I was filled with self-doubt; could I do justice to this story? Could anyone ever understand the destruction of lives? Our appointment was set for three o'clock, and at five to the hour I turned into her street. She lived in a quiet, middle-class community—split-level houses, well-kept gardens, primarily French-speaking. The house on the outside was pleasant but nondescript, with lace curtains at the picture window of what I assumed was the living room. As I mounted the steps my anxiety returned, and increased when I heard the barking of a rather large dog.

"*Lili, attends. Pas de bruits.*" The door opened, and a rather attractive middle-aged woman, grasping a large collie, appeared in the doorway. Her hair was cut in a young, carefree style, and she was dressed in a pretty blouse and pants that emphasized her slim figure. The blond hair framed a face that was striking for two reasons: first, because she looked younger than I thought her age to be; second, because her eyes were distinctly at variance with the rest of her features. They were eyes filled with pain; tiny lines at the corners showed resignation and fatigue. My father's eyes are like that, I thought. She smiled and, holding on to the dog, she invited me to come in.

"You are much younger than I thought you would be," she said. "How is your father?"

I looked around the room. While the outside of the house had looked well kept, the inside showed the strains of a pinched pocketbook. The living room furniture was old and in poor condition—the couch covered with a throw to hide the threadbare cushions. As she led me to a chair at the dining room table, I caught a glimpse of a bedroom on the next level; it was bare. The stark, empty room struck me as symbolic of the barren existence that Cameron's patients would have experienced when their sense of self was ripped away by the depatterning. Through the back window, I could see a small but pleasant garden surrounded by trees.

She apologized for the house and told me that, years ago, things had been much different. Once, money had been no problem—they had even owned a small place in the mountains—but now, all the amenities were gone. Her husband had become disabled and she was faced with increasing mortgage payments as she borrowed more to provide some income; she was still too young for a government pension. I explained to her what I was writing about and why I had wanted to talk to her. I had seen her on the television program "Sixty Minutes," the same segment for which I was interviewed. At that time, I had been struck by her poignant sadness, the yearning for normality.

She took a deep breath and said, heavily, that she did not know if she could talk. "When I think about all these things, it makes me so sad. I cannot do anything afterward." She looked down for a moment, and I felt a rush of sympathy. I asked her to try to tell me her story and assured her that I could understand because I had lived through a similar experience with my father for many years.

She was in her late fifties. Her parents were middle-class—her father was an electrician; her mother, a housewife. The only girl sandwiched between two brothers, she remembers her early years as being happy. She was born in Montreal, and when she reached adolescence, the family moved to the Laurentian Mountains for several years, during which time she blossomed. "I skied all the time. I was happy, filled with *joie de vivre*." After they returned to Montreal, she described a life filled with high school, friends, and dating. She entered business school and in her early twenties began to work in an office as a secretary. "Life was good. I had many friends. Oh, I was careful about whom I chose to be friendly with; they were nice girls. We went to parties, balls. Did you know Sir George Williams College? I went to the balls there." As she talked on, I could see her, almost thirty years ago, pretty and bubbling, a vivacious French-Canadian woman, filled with the impetuosity of youth, vain in the adolescent, narcissistic way, and filled with gossip of boys and clothes and make-up. She enjoyed working; her best job was policy-writing for an insurance company. Many of the people she knew then are still friends today.

In 1952, when she was twenty-two years old, she married her current husband, a businessman. She worked for two more years until she had the first of her four children. In 1957 the problems began, and she saw Dr. Cameron for the first time.

Her memory of these events is uncertain, but her story of treatment is consistent with what is known about the therapy at the Allan Memorial during those years.

"In 1957, shortly after my second child was born, I began to lose my hearing. I became very anxious and depressed and my sleep was affected because I was afraid that I would not hear my baby if she cried in the night. Things got worse when the baby got septicemia. She was very sick and had to go to the hospital." In 1957–58, she began treatment with Cameron as an outpatient. Shock treatments were administered and drugs were prescribed. She had been referred to Cameron by her family doctor and she continued to see him for the next five years. She notes that she never received psychotherapy; she saw Cameron as very authoritarian: "I was afraid of him. Isn't that funny?"

In 1958–59, Jeanine was hospitalized for depression. She again attributes her difficulties to the hearing loss. She was also anemic and weak, likely because of excessive bleeding during her menstrual periods, and she received blood transfusions during this time. She has little memory of that hospitalization. In 1961, following the birth of her last child, she was rehospitalized and given semi-sleep treatment plus insulin comas. She was then transferred to the day hospital where she received drugs with no names, "just numbers." Shortly thereafter, she was rehospitalized and given drugs, sleep treatment, and ECT. It was also at this time that psychic driving was begun.

"The nurse said to me, 'There's a machine over your head. You have to listen.' 'No,' I said, 'no way, no way. I'm not in Russia . . . no way.' " But the drugs, she said, made her give up the fight and she started to listen. The voice came through earphones; it was a male voice and very deep. What he was saying filled her with despair: " 'You are rejecting your family. . . . You're no good to your family.' "

"I thought that they wanted to drive me crazy. I found myself looking for paper on the floor and I didn't know why." This was a response to the driving cue that Cameron had developed to test the efficacy of the program: the statement would have been: "If you see a paper on the floor, pick it up." My father had received the same message.

Jeanine thinks that she received about seventeen or eighteen days of the negative driving messages. She became very suspicious and thought that she was being filmed by Cameron (and possibly she was). Nitrous oxide was administered because, "I didn't want to listen." She remembers that Cameron was very sharp to her; he would stop by for five minutes and then be off. Her husband could not obtain any information from Cameron despite the fact that the family was paying him and the hospital for the treatment.

At one point, the family became so concerned that, after her release on a pass, her husband and mother tried to keep her at home. The nurse threatened to call the police and the family backed down out of fear and ignorance. Jeanine continued to fight the voices; she tried to run away from the room and the machine. She remembers the voice of her doctor cajoling her—"Come on Jeanine, go back and listen." She knows that she was injected with curare, and she remembers other scattered but bizarre events. "There was a place behind the hospital. I think that they called it 'The Stables.' They did experiments on me there. They gave me injections; they blew air in my eyes. I think that the doctor was testing to see how much air I could stand in my eyes. I remember plastic glasses." The glasses were probably the goggles that were used as part of the technique to place patients in sensory isolation for driving. "One time, I was given an injection; the nurses got all distorted. . . . I was moving and moving."

The memories flowed as we talked. Dark shadows passed through her mind and onto her face. She struggled to control her feelings as she recounted the facts, as she recalled days and nights in a dim room with only a deep voice for company. The house was very quiet.

I commented that it must have been very difficult to try to raise a young family when she had been so drugged and disoriented. She sighed deeply and described how her mother had taken over the running of her house. Clearly this was the most painful aspect of the experience.

> I was a good mother but I couldn't be playful; I couldn't go on vacations or attend Christmas dinners. I couldn't go skiing with my children. All I could do was to stay cooped up in my house; I didn't want to see anyone. I felt guilty because my place was here and he kept me there. When my children were young, they wanted to play chess, and I could not. It was hard to be a mother because you need authority and I had none.

The subject of her children hurt her. She felt that all of them had been deeply affected by the years of illness, some more than others. She still could not come to terms with the feelings of guilt.

She did not see Cameron after 1962. She did not want to go back to him. Her mother lived with her for the next ten years, and for that entire time she sat and watched her mother cook and clean. Sadly, she notes that the downhill spiral, with its toll on her spirit and with the drain it imposed on the family finances, put great stress on the relationship with her husband. As with my family, the pebble once dropped into the pool created ripples that in ever-widening circles engulfed more and more family members, threatening to destroy all the structures that provide stability to family life.

In the early 1960s her hearing problem was diagnosed as otosclerosis, and surgery corrected the condition. At about this time, a new symptom appeared. She describes it as muscle paralysis or spasm. It would affect her legs, which would suddenly go out from under her; her face was affected as well, so she had to wear a scarf. Soon after, she went with her mother to the Mayo Clinic to try to uncover the origins of this condition. They were there for three days, and she says that the cause was never discovered: "I had these spasms for years." The history, although vague, suggests that the spasms may have been side effects of the drugs that she was taking.

Jeanine was rehospitalized in 1965–66, but life began to improve only in the 1970s: "I was hooked on drugs; afraid to have them. I don't want to go on that again."

Throughout the recounting of the story, she never cried: "I can't cry easily." I asked her to tell me what life was like for her now. She noted that she is plagued with problems in concentration; at times she becomes disoriented and, when walking outside, she loses track of direction, being unable to tell north from south. She also described an unusual symptom in that she is unable to recognize familiar people in different surroundings. Although I did not take a detailed neurological history, this could be a symptom of a central nervous system disturbance called prosopagnosia. Agnosia is a neurological term that refers to a disorder of recognition. It suggests that there is a disruption in the pathways of sensation and association, so that a familiar object or person cannot be identified. Usually, the disturbance lies in one sensory sphere such as the visual or auditory. In Jeanine's situation, the disturbance would appear to lie in the ability to recall or associate a face with the memory of a person when the context in which the person has been known changes. I knew that such a symptom had been reported by one of Cameron's other patients.

She experiences periods of great depression and anxiety but, for the most part, is able to carry on. She notes, however, that she cannot stand too much activity, and would rather be alone. Too many people make her moody and she then withdraws. Consequently, she is now always fighting a strong need to be cooped up, whereas at the Allan Memorial she was always fighting the fear of being confined. Her ability to socialize is also limited by her financial straits.

A short while ago, she decided to study to be a translator. Since she has a facility for language and is fluently bilingual in French and English, this seemed a reasonable course of action. But she began to develop migraine headaches; her ability to concentrate was so restricted that she could not study or take examinations. So she remains at home. She has some interests; she reads the newspapers and is current in world affairs. She loves nature, science, and all kinds of music. In the area of relationships, however, her psychological problems interfere. She now has grandchildren whom she dearly loves, but she cannot babysit because she becomes too anxious; she has no patience and does not want the children to feel that. Once again, as in my family, the effects are felt through three generations. Parent, child, grandchild—a dark cloud of sorrow and shame lies on all.

I asked Jeanine what sustained her. How did she keep going in the face of the pain that life had thrown her way? "I pray alone . . . I talk to God . . . I believe in God. . . ." She still has dreams—dreams of owning a greenhouse where she could tend her beloved flowers year round, and dreams of travel—to France, England—dreams of being free and open to adventure.

She no longer sees a psychiatrist. Her family doctor prescribes small amounts of antianxiety medication when she is under great stress. She lives with the hope that the court case against the CIA will be resolved in her favor, and that she will be able to pick up the pieces of her life.

Her son had been encouraging her to go to his cabin in the Laurentians for a week since her deposition to the CIA had resulted in significant depression. She could not make up her mind whether to go. Her home is her only security; to leave even for as short a time as a week is a threat. She worries that, as the money runs out, she may lose the house. I well understand what that would mean—the loss of our family's house was a pivotal point in my life.

As I rose to leave, she sat still for a moment and then wished me well. I felt a heaviness that all my years of working with depression, fear, and even craziness could not protect me against. I could not distance myself from her loss, and so, to my surprise, our talk was as hard on me as it must have been on her.

The warm summer afternoon washed over me as I walked down the steps. Two little girls were skipping rope. A delivery truck was moving a new bed into the house across the street. I drove back to Montreal and I cried.

12

The Story of Dr. Mary Morrow: The Pain of a Physician

Montreal, early on a summer morning, is a beautiful city. Trees and flowers are everywhere, and the combination of old stone buildings and tree-lined streets lends a gracious elegance to the French metropolis. I had decided to talk with one other of Cameron's patients; in many ways, this woman held a special fascination for me because she herself was a psychiatrist, and she had been fighting to rectify the injustice of her situation for more than ten years. She now lived in a small town in eastern Ontario on the New York border, and it was going to take me the better part of a day to drive there.

The brilliance of the sunshine in the streets of Westmount contrasted sharply with the gloom that I felt inside. The process of learning how the events at the Allan had affected people's lives was draining and frightening. I had become increasingly aware that I was always perturbed, usually lost in thought; part of me was fixed in the past, making connections and trying to understand. This withdrawal was affecting my sons, who had on the evening before accused me of no longer paying enough attention to them. When I reached the highway leading toward Toronto, I tried to listen to some music, but I soon switched it off. My thoughts were overwhelming in their push for exploration, and so I succumbed to the luxury of several hours of framing my thoughts about the people I had met who were somehow involved with Cameron.

Dr. Mary Morrow's letter to me had been very cordial; she was planning to take the afternoon off, and indeed had invited me to lunch with her. She would not be unfamiliar to me since she too had taken part in the television program "Sixty Minutes," and I had been struck then with her determination and strength. The next day when I reached her town, I began to follow the directions on the hand-drawn map that she had thoughtfully provided. The town looked as though it had a population of about twenty-five thousand, and it was located along a river valley that combined farms and forests with glimpses of the wide and inviting water. The town itself was a mixture of old Victorian houses, modern motels, and fast-food places. I drove through the streets into a newer subdivision that was hilly, well landscaped, and bordered on forest. Most of the houses were ranch style except for one two-story, brick, and gabled structure: this was the home and office of Dr. Morrow. It was a pretty house on a pleasant cul-de-sac, and, I thought, it looked substantial and secure. As I reached the front door, it opened, and two women stood in the doorway. The older wished the younger well and indicated that she would see her next week; it was the end of a patient's visit. The doctor then turned to me, and, with a big smile, welcomed me in. She was dressed very stylishly in a lively summer frock; her hair was worn in a youthful cut and had been colored to an auburn shade; her make-up was skillfully applied, and, indeed, her overall appearance was that of a lively and exuberant woman. She was much shorter than I am, and her active movements made me think of a little bird hopping about as she ushered me into her office.

She began to talk almost at once, and I remember thinking that she seemed genuinely happy to have someone there with whom she could discuss the lawsuit. She was clearly very proud of both her house and the office—she showed me the waiting area and then the living room, and offered me a seat. It was a pleasant room, decorated in warm reds and oranges. She, too, was in red and white—she seemed to surround herself with happy colors. A wall of bookcases lined one side of the room containing the latest works in adolescent psychiatry, depression, psychopharmacology, and short-term psychotherapy. Recent journals were also neatly displayed. On her desk was one pen and a notepad. I was struck by the contrast with my own desk and its sloppy piles of unfinished projects. On the walls hung diplomas and certificates, fellowships and residency completion documents. The office was very professional—it showed care and thought for patient comfort, and was clearly the work of someone who wanted to instill a sense of ease. The sterile work of a high-tech decorator was not part of the impression that she was trying to create.

We began to discuss her recent deposition to the CIA. Her righteous indignation filled the room as she described how the attorney for the CIA had compared her and the other plaintiffs to the mice with which she had once worked at the National Institutes of Health in Washington, D.C. This anger toward those who did not in her eyes respect her humanity, her dignity as a human being, was to emerge repeatedly during the course of the several hours that we spent together. She began to tell me a little about herself.

Mary Morrow was born in Montreal sixty-nine years ago, one of three children, to a cardiologist father and a mother whose background was in nursing. Her older brother is an economist; her younger sister, a nurse. She grew up fairly close to McGill University where her father taught in the medical school. Carrying on the family tradition of involvement with medicine, Mary graduated from medical school at McGill in the early 1950s. In fact, as we talked, it was apparent that her identity as a physician, her commitment to the ideals of the Hippocratic oath, and her need to be professionally competent lie at the core of what has sustained her through the years.

Following graduation, she completed a residency in neurology at the University of Michigan in Ann Arbor, and studied further at the New England Deaconess Hospital in Boston. She returned to Montreal in the mid-1950s, and for four or five years was in practice in neurology at a local hospital where she was also the director of the neurology clinic. She was not doing as well financially as she would have liked, and so she thought that she would become a psychiatrist and specialize as one of the few neuropsychiatrists in the area. She approached Ewen Cameron at the Allan Memorial in December 1959 for a fellowship. The legal complaint filed in United States District Court in Washington, D.C., outlines what then transpired:

> Because Cameron thought she appeared "nervous," he told Dr. Morrow that a medical examination would be required before her application could be considered. Dr. Morrow was then hospitalized at the Royal Victoria Hospital, a facility affiliated with McGill University and the Allan Memorial Institute. After she left the Royal Victoria Hospital, Dr. Morrow was admitted as a paying patient at the Allan Memorial Institute on May 6, 1960, and placed under Cameron's care. For an eleven day period from May 19, 1960, through May 29, 1960, Dr. Morrow was subjected to depatterning experiments employing Page-Russell electroconvulsive shock treatments and a variety of barbiturates, specifically thorazine and anectine [*sic*]. The combination of these drugs produced a condition of brain anoxia [insufficient oxygen reaching the brain] in Dr. Morrow and on June 17, 1960, she was transferred, at her family's insistence, to the medical department of the Royal Victoria Hospital, where she was diagnosed as suffering from acute laryngeal edema [a severe allergic reaction to the experimental combination of drugs she had received].

Mary's father had died when she was younger, so only her mother was around at that time to be of assistance. Unfortunately, her mother had suffered a stroke shortly before and could not leave the house. When Mary entered the hospital, her mother called daily to check on her condition; she became increasingly concerned about the rapid deterioration in Mary's ability to communicate and called her other daughter who was in New York to return to Montreal and assist Mary.

Margie, Mary's younger sister, telephoned Cameron at his home in Lake Placid and demanded that Mary either be discharged or the treatment ended. He countered by saying that Mary was no good and he washed his hands of her treatment. The sister also called the hospital and informed them that she would call the police if this "treatment" did not end at once. By that time, the thorazine was causing severe central nervous system side effects, and shortly thereafter, Mary developed an acute swelling of the larynx that was life threatening. Following emergency treatment at the Royal Victoria Hospital, she left for home. Like other victims of Cameron, Mary was left with neurological damage. As she reported on "Sixty Minutes," she suffers from prosopagnosia—a disorder of recognition.

While in the hospital, Mary threatened to institute a lawsuit, and, beginning in 1962, she began following through with this threat; legal involvement continued into the 1970s. She notes that when she consulted with other physicians, "they thought I was a crazy woman" and would not consider her story valid. All of this changed greatly when *The Search for the Manchurian Candidate* was published in 1979.

After the hospitalization in 1960–61, Mary tried to pick up the pieces of her life, but her struggle for self-worth was only beginning. She went to St. Louis to the Missouri Institute of Psychiatry to do a residency in psychiatry. This was a state hospital, and the criteria for admission would have been less strict at that point than those at medical schools; her history of hospitalization would not then have jeopardized her application. She completed the residency training program in psychiatry and applied to take the examinations of the American Board of Psychiatry. To her great surprise, she was turned down because her "references were no good." She then tried to pursue her career by taking a series of state hospital jobs, finally coming to work at a hospital in New York State close to the border with Canada, where she functioned as a neurologist as well as a psychiatrist.

During the course of attempting to gather evidence for

the lawsuit against the Royal Victoria Hospital, she discovered that Cameron had written to the American Board claiming that she was "too crazy" to be a psychiatrist. Encouraged by one of the psychiatrists who was testifying for her, she reapplied to take the examinations, and was finally permitted to do so.

In the late 1970s, she moved across the border to the town where she currently resides. By that time, she had passed the certifying examinations of the Royal College in Canada and was licensed to practice medicine in two provinces and one state. She worked at the local general hospital for a short while, but by then was sixty-five years old, and was forced to leave because of her age. She also began a private practice and continued to work part time at the state hospital in New York. Currently, she continues in practice, and works one half-day a week as a neurologist.

I was deeply moved by this woman's struggle to achieve her professional position. Dr. Morrow had spent years in her quest to become a psychiatrist. Against many odds, she had triumphed, but the cost had been high. As she talked, the underlying tone was that of suppressed rage—anger at Cameron and the Royal Victoria, anger at those who had impeded her progress, hurt and frustration with those who offered to help and then disappointed her.

At that point in our conversation, she suggested that we go out to lunch. She had arranged for our meal at a local restaurant and she insisted on driving. On arrival, it was clear that she had checked out the menu and arranged to pay for the lunch beforehand. I was very touched and impressed at her need to take full control of the situation and, most specifically, with her vivid demonstration to me that she was a capable human being. I was certain that she carried on the rest of her life in this same fashion, working hard to show her strengths and never allowing anyone to see weakness or vulnerability.

Over "Shrimp Louis" and wine, she was affable and open as we discussed a variety of topics. She had been a physician for more than thirty-five years and she planned to continue until she was unable physically to go on. Medicine was her life and she was proud of her competence as a doctor. She said that neurology was her first love, but it was readily apparent that she was very well-versed in psychiatry as well.

After lunch, we returned to her home and continued our discussion in the garden. Gradually, she revealed aspects of her life that demonstrated the profound impact that the hospitalization had on her. The anger that she hinted at earlier began to emerge more clearly.

"Humiliation and stigma, that's what I feel, not guilt." She was concerned about publicity because she is a professional woman. She felt that people would think less of her if they knew what she went through. She had been battling this humiliation for years and felt very alone in the fight. There was no one to talk with about the case; she was concerned that even her sister might be bored with the topic. And then she told me how sad her life was; she has her house, a garden, and her puppy, but is isolated. She complained that she had not been permitted to participate actively in the life of the medical community in which she lives. She is a member of all the major medical organizations, but not her local society. She reported that, for a long time, they would not consider her. During the last year, she had tried once again and received a message on her answering machine that she was invited to the next social function. When she went, her discomfort was so great that she never returned.

There were two other psychiatrists in the town. She never saw them or received any referrals from them. She had no referrals from any of the physicians in the area, and yet she was, she believed, highly thought of at the state hospital. She became feisty and overtly angry as she described this professional isolation: "I don't see myself as successful as I could have been." She feels that she has been exiled to this little town trying to make a go of the rest of her life. She expressed bitterness and frustration with medical professionals and psychiatrists, whom she sees as arrogant and power crazy.

Her dilemma revolves around the fact that medicine is her life; it is her principal identification. Yet medicine has done her in—she has been physically hurt, emotionally attacked, and professionally rejected. She is thus left with profound ambivalence and an insoluble internal conflict that winning a lawsuit will surely not resolve. Her ambivalence toward the medical profession rang a bell inside me, for my whole professional life has been dedicated to the resolution of a similar conflict.

I looked around the garden—the white lawn furniture, the trees and blooming flowers, the house so comfortable and filled with all the furniture and appliances one could ask for, the late model car in which we had driven to lunch. I thought of Jeanine Huard and the empty room, the shabby furniture. I pictured my father, smoking alone in a tiny apartment. All three fight against an emptiness inside, a void that was opened many years ago when part of themselves was torn away. On the outside, Dr. Morrow seemed so much a success, but she, too, was one of the walking wounded.

As I looked at the photograph of Mary's medical school class, I was struck at the difference in her appearance. The changes seemed to me to be more than those due to age, and I wondered at the extent to which the shock treatments and thorazine had ravaged her. She kept in touch with some of her classmates, but felt that most saw her as a maverick. She had gone to her last class reunion but doubted that she would attend another.

The afternoon passed as we talked. It was pleasant in her garden, and I was charmed by her sense of humor; intermixed with the very real bitterness was an ability to smile at herself. As she thought about the case in Washington, it seemed to evoke for her all the pain that she had experienced in trying to obtain retribution. She felt that the Canadian lawyers had let her down in the past. She had spent thousands of dollars in her quest for justice, and was still repaying this debt. As we discussed medical politics, I realized that the two groups that most aroused her ire were the two on whom she was most dependent—doctors and lawyers.

We began to discuss our clinical experience with various of our patients. I realized as I asked about some diagnostic dilemmas that I was testing her, trying to ascertain if she were really a good psychiatrist. How presumptuous of me!

And yet, I was caught in the web of stigma. She was right to be concerned about how others viewed her, because I had no valid reason to question her competence. This realization made me both ashamed and very sad, because it meant that Cameron's handiwork on this woman had influenced me. In fact, she was thoughtful and sensitive. She took on difficult patients and worked hard for them. She impressed me as a genuinely caring physician.

I wanted to set out for Montreal before the end of the day, so our discussion drew to a close. She walked me to the front door and stood there as I drove off. She seemed almost frail then, and I felt guilty for seeing her this way because I was sure that she would find it most unacceptable.

When I think about Dr. Morrow, I picture a woman who has been left with both physical and emotional consequences of her "treatment." Her personality has been so affected that she might appear to be both eccentric and angry. It is, however, her anger and feistiness that have made her quite competent to take care of herself. She prizes independence and finds it difficult to be part of any group (such as the plaintiffs against the CIA), but she feels cut, wounded to the quick, because she feels that she does not belong anywhere. She lives with a sense of isolation and failure.

I believe that her life would have been very different if the events of 1960 had not occurred, if Cameron had not stood in her way. Perhaps she would have been in academic medicine or in a private practice in a major metropolitan area, a situation more closely resembling her dream. I drove away from our encounter feeling enormous respect for this colleague. I had somehow expected to find a professional failure, but discovered instead a woman who had tenaciously fought her way past enormous obstacles to achieve many of her career goals. It felt good to realize that human dignity can triumph. During the course of that afternoon, she gave me strength.

Part 3: The Fight

13

Learning the Law

Strength was only part of what I needed. As the months passed after the "Sixty Minutes" show, I began to wish that I had taken a degree in law. Fighting the CIA meant taking on all the resources of the United States government. Submissions, countersubmissions, waiting for decisions—and the years flew by.

The pursuit of justice is complex and, at times, excruciatingly slow. The courtroom drama is but the end result of months, even years, of painstaking preparation by attorneys. A process takes place that is called "pretrial discovery." This involves the gathering of evidence and the taking of depositions from the principal characters in order to record their stories. Often, attempts are made to settle the case by negotiation before it reaches the courtroom while, at the same time, the defending side may be attempting to have the case thrown out on one legal ground or another. The wheels of law grind at a slow pace, and as they do, the characters in the drama grow older and older.

I would like to describe our search for justice by an examination of some of the documents that have been filed with the court, as well as by a consideration of some of the key events that have modified the course of the case. Clearly, I must draw primarily upon the plaintiffs' view of their experiences and ultimately it is for the court to decide on the validity of facts and allegations. However, this process is of value because the case raises issues that go far beyond the concerns of the nine plaintiffs involved. Issues of medical experimentation, intelligence and secrecy, the relationship between Canada and the United States, and the importance of human decency are all involved in the events of the last few years.

Several themes have consistently emerged since the case was filed in 1980. First, the CIA has refused to accept any responsibility whatsoever for the work that was carried out in Montreal. Its position is that Cameron was not carrying out research, but was only doing his best for the patients, that his work utilized approaches that were standard for that time, and that the consents obtained from the patients were acceptable according to those same standards. On another front, the political maneuverings of the Government of Canada with respect to the United States have proven to be a puzzling aspect of the case.

From the earliest communications of the CIA to our lawyers, Joe Rauh and Jim Turner, the CIA has disavowed responsibility for Subproject 68 of their MKULTRA mind-control project (Cameron's work). They have asserted that Cameron approached the Society for the Investigation of Human Ecology (the CIA front) with an unsolicited proposal to carry out the research on depatterning and psychic driving. But in January 1983, John W. Gittinger, the CIA psychologist who had functioned as the project monitor for the Society on Subproject 68, testified in his deposition that the proposal from Ewen Cameron had been solicited by Colonel James Monroe, the executive secretary of the Society, at his behest. This reaching out by the CIA to develop projects that would enhance its knowledge of mind control appears to be consistent with what is known about MKULTRA.

The abrogation of responsibility, which has been the CIA's response to this case up to the present, flies in the face of what had been known CIA policy. When Admiral Stansfield Turner, who was then Director of Central Intelligence, provided testimony before the joint hearing of the Select Committee on Intelligence and the Subcommittee on Health and

Scientific Research of the Committee on Human Resources of the United States Senate in August 1977, the chairman of the Intelligence Committee, Senator Daniel Inouye of Hawaii, stated:

> A sad aspect of the MKULTRA project was that it naturally involved the people who unwittingly or wittingly got involved in experimentation. I would appreciate it if you would report back to this committee in three months on what the Agency has done to notify these individuals and these institutions, and furthermore, to notify us as to what steps have been taken to identify victims, and if identified, what you have done to assist them, monetarily or otherwise.

In response, Turner stated, "All right, sir, I will be happy to." No patients of Subproject 68 were ever contacted. Turner's statement was an empty promise to a committee that would not follow through on its request.

Yet the CIA's irresponsibility had been part and parcel of its involvement with MKULTRA from the beginning. As has been well described elsewhere, the tragic death of Frank Olson was a direct result of the reckless manipulations of those responsible for the agency's mind-control work. In November 1953, Drs. Sidney Gottlieb and Robert Lashbrook secretly administered LSD to a group of CIA-affiliated scientists of the Army Chemical Corps at a rural retreat in Maryland. One of those men, Dr. Frank Olson, an employee of the U.S. Army, began to experience profound and serious effects of the drug; he became increasingly paranoid, agitated, and depressed. He was subsequently taken to New York City by Lashbrook to see a CIA-associated physician, and leaped to his death in the middle of the night from a hotel window.

Despite the findings of the Inspector General of the CIA, Lyman Kirkpatrick, and General Counsel Lawrence Houston, Gottlieb and Lashbrook were not even reprimanded. Gottlieb continued in his role with MKULTRA as chief of the CIA's chemical division and became the Agency officer who approved the funding for Ewen Cameron two years later. It appears that, despite what is known about the extensive and dangerous nature of the MKULTRA projects, the CIA has never recognized its responsibility for the potential (and actual) destruction of the human mind.

There have been some indications of worry on the agency's part. William Allard, the assistant to the CIA general counsel, wrote that "the substantial funds flowing from this Agency to McGill in support of the project subsequent to 1956 would appear to preclude the determination that this Agency was minimally involved," that "long-term after-effects may have been involved," and that "it is doubtful that any meaningful form of consent is involved in this case." Stansfield Turner testified on deposition that the MKULTRA experiments on unwitting individuals were "unethical" and left him "aghast." Gittinger, in his deposition, described his views on the CIA's involvement with Cameron as follows:

> Now that was a foolish mistake. We shouldn't have done it. . . . As I said, I'm sorry we did it. Because it turned out to be a terrible mistake. . . . I think there were a lot of things that probably were wrong with this, but they were not things that I knew anything about. And I am basing this on what I know after the fact.

If he had to do it over, "I would refuse to support him or be interested in him."

During the spring of 1984, Allan MacEachen, the external affairs minister for the Government of Canada, revealed to David Orlikow, the member of Parliament whose wife had been a patient of Cameron, that in the late 1970s the United States had apologized to Canada for the CIA's funding of Cameron and had promised that nothing like that would ever happen again. Clearly, this was an admission of culpability, and attempts were made by Rauh and Turner to obtain copies of any documents that were relevant to this action. Both the American and the Canadian governments refused to release any specific documents concerning the apologies.

During 1983 and 1984, attempts were made to negotiate an out-of-court settlement. In January 1984, the CIA offered to settle the dispute on a "nuisance" basis and offered $15,000 to $20,000 per plaintiff. Not surprisingly, this offer was rejected. At the end of 1984, the new external affairs minister, Joe Clark, stated that the Canadian government had received a signal from the United States that they wished to pursue settlement negotiations. The attorneys then reduced the claim considerably and waited for the CIA response. Once again, deception appeared to be the game since no new offer appeared. Instead, the same "nuisance" number was advanced. What I think is significant in all of this is how the Canadian government was either taken in by the game or else was cooperating with the United States in a process of wearing down the case of the nine Canadians.

The issue of whether the United States had indeed apologized became critical at this point. For indeed, apology would be an admission of culpability. The two CIA station chiefs in Ottawa during the 1970s had been previously identified in several publications as two men named John Kenneth Knaus and Stacey Hulse; therefore, their identities were no longer secret. The Canadian intelligence liaison, John Hadwen, had publicly stated that he had met with a representative of the United States Embassy in September 1977 regarding the issue of CIA funding to the Allan Memorial Institute. At that meeting, the Canadian government had expressed its disapproval of CIA funding within Canada of experimental procedures without prior approval of the government. The two American intelligence men were contacted by the attorneys and both agreed to give depositions. The CIA then refused to allow them to do so. The issue went before the judge based on the alleged security concerns of the CIA over a compromise of their "sources and methods."

The judge ruled that the CIA had the right to keep the activities of the two station agents secret, and in addition, he denied the request to order the CIA to make public documents about the apologies. His conclusion was based upon a decision of the Supreme Court of the United States in April 1985, in which the court decided that the CIA did not have to disclose the names of some of the 185 private researchers who participated in the MKULTRA experiments. In his ruling, Judge John Penn of the United States District Court of the District of Columbia said: "Courts do not have sufficient background or expertise to formulate a knowledgeable decision as to what may be harmful to the intelligence-gathering procedures used by this country or helpful to other countries."

I had been very concerned when I had read the newspaper accounts of that Supreme Court ruling in April. I then wrote a letter to the *San Francisco Chronicle* conveying my dismay about the decision—a letter that they chose not to print. I wrote:

> Through the Freedom of Information Act, nine of these patients were able to obtain enough information to finally learn what happened to them—to learn that the CIA had funded experiments on innocent Canadian citizens—not terrorists or subversives, but people who were living routine law-abiding lives. If the Supreme Court ruling had been in effect, this would not have been known. How sad that the arrogance of government will prevail; that the lessons of the 1950s and 1960s will be so easily lost.

Consequently, information that might have been helpful was no longer available.

In May 1985, I was giving a paper at a meeting in Washington, D.C., and for the first time I had the opportunity to meet Jim Turner and Joe Rauh. I was both excited and not a little in awe as I entered the building where their law office was located. The suite was plain and unprepossessing, in a building that was utilitarian. A large central waiting room also held the desks of two secretaries. Off the room were four other offices. Clearly, this was not the luxury of corporate law, the 350-person firm. It was a masculine environment—mementos, photographs—the personality of its senior partner clearly dominated the setting. Jim came out to greet me. Thin, bearded, about my height and probably somewhat younger than me, he was very genial, and I felt quite comfortable with him. He ushered me into "Joe's office." It was a spacious corner room with light flooding in from two sides. A sturdy conference table with massive chairs dominated one side of the room; at the far end stretched a long desk. The walls were covered with photographs and honorary degrees: Lyndon Johnson, John Kennedy, Supreme Court justices, an honorary degree from the Hebrew Union College. The room was a striking embodiment of its owner. It reflected a long career, prestigious colleagues, the esteem of many. The impression was of enormous vitality and force.

Joe Rauh rose from behind the desk as I entered the office. He was very tall, over six feet, silver-haired, and slightly portly. Impeccably dressed, he portrayed the image of a Washington lawyer very well. The booming voice was friendly, but by then, I felt as though I was six years of age and incapable of speaking in a coherent fashion. I suppose that, in retrospect, it was the vigor and drive that was so overwhelming. We went to a restaurant for lunch—Rauh, Turner, Mary Levy (another partner in the firm), and I. Over the meal, I discussed my father's story, answering the precise questions that were directed at me.

Toward the end of the meal, they revealed some plans that they had in mind for me. First, they wanted me to see Alan Gotlieb, the Canadian ambassador to the United States; second, they suggested that I grant interviews to the media, specifically the Canadian press and the *Washington Post*. I had, at their behest, appeared on "Sixty Minutes" several months earlier. At that time, I had decided to overcome my natural shyness in order to assist the development of the case by public exposure. Now I was hesitant, but after further discussion I agreed to try to obtain an appointment with Ambassador Gotlieb, and to try to interest a *Post* reporter in the story.

I called the embassy from their office. The ambassador was not in town; several other staffers were offered as alternatives. Turner and Rauh had been working with another senior member of the embassy staff in trying to learn about the American apology to Canada. They suggested that I try to see him. After some haggling with embassy secretaries, it was arranged that I should call the embassy the next day. That afternoon, I called David Remnick of the *Washington Post* to try to interest him in the story. We arranged to meet, and at four o'clock I entered the lobby of the *Post*. I went up to Remnick's area and found myself in the heart of one of the most respected newspapers in the United States.

Here is where the Watergate story broke, I thought. By this time, I was feeling terribly anxious and somewhat detached from my surroundings. I was filled with disbelief that I was exposing myself and our family history to a newspaper.

After having my photograph taken, I returned to my hotel to face another interview with Norma Greenaway of the Canadian press. During the course of that interview, I finally broke down; the tears erupted from deep inside as I reacted to the strain that I had been under the whole day. I must say that, in retrospect, Norma and David were undoubtedly the most professional and thoughtful reporters with whom I have talked during the course of this case. I am grateful, because my experiences with them allowed me to become more confident in dealing with the media—a confidence that would be sorely tried in the succeeding months.

The following day, I telephoned the embassy and spoke with the official, Jeremy Kinsman. He was curt, but invited me to spend a short time with him. Canadians are characteristically imbued with a great reverence for government authority. For me, as I entered the magnificent old building that then housed the Canadian embassy offices on Massachusetts Avenue, I was once again amazed at my audacity. Who was I to try to enlist the support of the Canadian government against the power tactics of the United States?

Mr. Kinsman's office was immense, imposing, with high ceilings. He was elegant, a career diplomat. His friendly, smooth demeanor was a relief, but it also made me wonder if he could be trusted. What secrets was he capable of hiding? Once again, I told my story. He was interested and well informed. He told me that the CIA was insisting that the Canadian government was primarily responsible for Cameron's work, and had funded it to a considerably greater degree than had the Americans. The Canadian government was going to try to investigate this claim. As we talked, I felt that I could trust him, and I left the embassy with the sense that, perhaps, my own government would not let us down.

Much of the work on the case now seemed to revolve around the attempt to push the Canadian government to take responsibility for its citizens. The lawyers communicated directly with the Canadian government and I myself wrote to the external affairs minister, Joe Clark, asking him to intervene directly. Clark replied that he was indeed interested in the case, and considered it a matter of highest priority. He said that he had discussed it with George Shultz, then U.S. Secretary of State, at a meeting in May 1984. Unfortunately, private discussions are not a measure of strong concern in the area of international diplomacy. At this time, Joe Rauh was publicly stating that Canada should take the case to arbitration in the World Court at The Hague. Clark's response (as reported in the *Montreal Gazette*): "He doesn't want to refer the case of nine Canadians . . . to the World Court because the court's proceedings are slow and it doesn't have the power to award compensation to individuals." This, after five full years of foot-dragging in the American court system.

In any event, after meeting with Clark, Shultz had asked his legal advisor, Judge Abraham Sofaer, to review the case, and to advise him of appropriate direction. Judge Sofaer declined to meet with Rauh and Turner to review their documentation, and issued a report that, while denying the American government's liability, concluded that American courts should decide the merits of the case.

In the autumn of 1985, Clark and Shultz were again scheduled to meet in Calgary. I wrote an open letter to them asking that further consideration be given to a speedy resolution of the case, with a plea to Clark that Canada be more assertive in demanding a just solution. At the conclusion of that meeting, Canada was invited to send representatives to Washington to sift through files related to the brainwashing lawsuit. As noted in the *Montreal Gazette*: "A State Department official in Washington said the Shultz invitation is aimed at giving the Canadian Justice Department an opportunity 'to better understand our theory of the case—our view of the facts.' " Since Canada was still sitting on documents of its own related to the "apology" that was supposed to have been tendered to Canada, it is unclear who was hiding what from whom. What was becoming quite apparent, however, was the distinct lack of support emerging from the Government of Canada.

During the summer of 1985, I had written a piece for the *Toronto Globe and Mail* in which I demanded that the Canadian government become more active. Others were working on this problem as well. The attorneys were not only dealing with the issues before the judge but were also besieged with the machinations of the two governments. At that point, Canada was playing the part of the pristine virgin who has suffered an inadvertent deflowering by her best boyfriend. The United States government was the innocent and wounded friend, seductively inviting Canada to see how pure it was. Each was hiding documentation, and likely the truth, from each other.

In August 1985, Jeremy Kinsman, the senior Canadian embassy official with whom I had met in Washington, visited Stanford University to give a talk. He contacted me and we spent an hour together. He filled me in on what was transpiring between the governments and assured me that he would call in September or October as more was learned. I left our talk with the feeling that I could really trust him, that he was supportive of our attempts to obtain documentation that would reveal the truth. I never heard from him again.

In November, I telephoned the Canadian Embassy and learned, to my great surprise, that he had been transferred back to Canada, to a department and a position that had nothing to do with the foreign service. I could only hope that his interest and support had nothing to do with this sudden move. But I wondered.

During the autumn of 1985 I gave talks; I gave radio and television interviews; I talked to newspaper reporters. I began to have difficulty sleeping, as I would awaken filled with anger and helplessness. I could not talk with my father about all that I was doing, and my sisters had their hands full providing him with support. Friends were interested, but the intensity of the emotional involvement and the energy required to effect some movement in the process of resolution were uniquely mine. It was abundantly clear that, where a case involves events that are some thirty years old, the interest of the public is not readily sustained.

In desperation, I wrote the two senators from California, where I live. Senator Wilson replied: "I understand your concern and will be happy to initiate an inquiry on your behalf with the United States Central Intelligence Agency. As soon as I receive any information I will be in touch with you." A year passed, and I heard nothing. Senator Cranston also suggested that he could look into the situation, and I even received a follow-up call. A year later, nothing had happened. Tom Lantos, a local congressman, wrote: "This organization should be held accountable for its actions. We in Congress must make sure that the CIA's methods of obtaining information are reasonable and that they are justified by the importance of the results. In your father's case it seems that neither of these criteria have been met." He went on, however, to say: "This immediate circumstance is out of Congressional jurisdiction and must be settled in the courts." Senators Metzenbaum of Ohio and Dodd of Connecticut did not reply to my letters.

In the early months of 1986, international diplomacy, politics, and psychiatry began to merge in an arena of increasing hostility. Canada's External Affairs Minister Clark refused to meet with Joe Rauh in Ottawa. An exchange of letters between Prime Minister Brian Mulroney and Rauh revealed radically differing perceptions, both of the goodwill of the Canadian government and of its ability to be of assistance to its own citizens. I felt a surge of helplessness as the players strutted about the stage. The culmination was to be a report prepared for the Government of Canada, the so-called Cooper Report, that was to abandon nine people to their fate.

14

Psychiatry and Politics

As the months flew by, and events piled one on top of another, many of my long-held beliefs were to be called into question. For fifteen years, a major aspect of how I defined myself lay in my professional role of psychiatrist. Suddenly, I was forced to confront an ugliness, a shameful period of my profession's history that, when exposed to scrutiny, was either being ignored or excused. How could a respected member of the medical profession, a fellow psychiatrist, have undertaken such an endeavor? Not only that, how indeed could his colleagues not only have failed to question his judgment but have actually rewarded him for contributions to the field? Their silence gave him tacit permission to escalate the research; his techniques became increasingly more intrusive; the hapless patients found themselves at the mercy of a misguided and powerful enemy disguised as a healer. What did this mean about me? How could I comfortably wear the identity of psychiatrist? Did I still subscribe to all that I had learned over the last years?

My faith was to be further shaken as I observed the Government of Canada in ignominious retreat before the bravado of the CIA and its attorneys. My identity as a Canadian, an aspect of myself to which I had clung for the eighteen years since I had moved to the United States, was now in disarray. As I read the briefs, as I turned to Washington politicians for assistance and found no interest, my belief in American justice was gradually shattered. What was left for me to hold on to?

If I could make sense of the historical context, if I could understand the political currents that could create a program like MKULTRA, and a man like Ewen Cameron, would more pieces fall into place? Would that lessen the pain? And so I began to read—about America in the 1950s, about Canada as a nation, about psychiatry and politics.

During the 1940s, the psychiatric profession demonstrated its capabilities by effectively developing methods to handle the acute stress reactions of soldiers at the front. Many of the psychiatrists who contributed so much during the war became advisors to the postwar government. Patriotism was high, and psychiatrists, like most Americans, felt called upon to serve their country. During the 1950s and 1960s, psychiatry moved beyond its roots in biology, and indeed, beyond the psychodynamic legacy of Freud, to address the social conflicts of society. We began to hear more about the social and behavioral sciences, and psychiatric literature began to address issues of poverty and racism.

In retrospect, it is not surprising that eminent psychiatrists became involved in the work of the CIA and the United States Army, Navy, and Air Force. The driving force of the 1950s was patriotism; the intellectual challenge was mind control—changing the way that people think, and ultimately act. Funding allowed psychiatrists to pursue an understanding of how the brain actually worked. It is possible that, for many of these psychiatrists, the motivation was knowledge; but for others, especially those who were aware of the sources of funding and the specific interests of those agencies, one can only surmise that loyalty to their country pushed them on.

Another pervasive force in the United States during the early 1950s was a great fear and mistrust of the "Red Menace." The Russians, allies during World War II, had rapidly become the threatening bear of the following decade. At the same time, the Korean War, fought against a people who were so different physically, provoked significant fear in Americans. And then there was Senator Joe McCarthy. The profound impact he had on American society can barely be appreciated by those who did not live in the United States at that time.

A perusal of *The New York Times* during the early 1950s reveals the suspicion, fear, and hatred that marked the public mind.

> *March 11, 1952:*
> "Allies Bag 7 MIGS"
> "Red Danger Seen in East Pakistan"
> "Anti-Red Witness is Hazy on Dates"
> "Reds Burned Papers, FBI Informer Says"
> "Powers to Deport Red Aliens Upheld"
>
> *April 12, 1953:*
> "News Group Denies It Was Soviet Dupe"
> "Teacher Tenure Is Issue on Coast: Move to Change State Laws Arises as Witnesses Balk at House Red Queries"
>
> *February 21, 1954:*
> "True Unity Urged Against Red Foe"
> "College Papers Warned: Queens Student Council Bans Ads of Subversive Groups"
>
> *June 1, 1953:*
> "McCarthy Praised as Reds Opponent"

It was in this hysterical climate that the idea of being brainwashed evolved. The brainwashing methodology developed by Edward Hunter, the CIA, and the military could easily be used to attract eminent psychiatrists to the task of both understanding how one could gain control of another human being and, in addition, protect oneself against such control. Thus, Harold Wolff, Harold Abramson, Lawrence Hinkle, Harris Isbell, Carl Pfeiffer, James Hamilton, and others who received money from the coffers of MKULTRA could pursue their own professional interests and meet their country's needs as well.

In Canada, the impact of the Cold War was less intense.

The revelation shortly after the war that a defecting Russian clerk by the name of Igor Gouzenko had been assisted by Canadian citizens in passing secret files to the Russians did lead to a national awareness of espionage as a postwar fact of life. However, as John Holmes, an eminent Canadian foreign policy expert, has noted:

> We were less inclined to attribute all revolutionary activity, especially in Asia, to Moscow's direction and we regarded that continent as a very complex area of the world. Communism as an ideology was certainly not regarded with a friendly eye in Ottawa, but the objections were more liberal than capitalist. It was the threatening behavior of communist states and their denial of the human rights of even their own citizens rather than their discredited economics which drove Canada into hostility. . . . Canadians might in retrospect be called premature detentistes.

Canadian patriotism has always been a far more subtle theme than the flag-waving fireworks of the United States. Yet Canada, too, was touched at an official level by theories of brainwashing. It is known that in 1951 a meeting took place at the Ritz Carlton Hotel in Montreal. Present were representatives of Canada, the United States, and Britain; of the two Americans in the room, one was an admitted CIA operative, the other was likely a CIA agent as well. They were doubtless seeking information for the newly established Project Artichoke. As a result of that meeting, Donald Hebb received his initial funding for the sensory deprivation work that was to be taken up by the United States within the next few years. That said, however, it does appear that the Canadian mental health establishment, unlike its American counterpart, did not adopt mind control as an area of serious research.

And so psychiatry and politics had merged their interests in the United States and, to a lesser extent, in Canada as well. To me, that was startling and deeply disturbing. What further shocked me out of my naiveté was something I learned in 1986—that international politics can play a significant role in influencing a search for truth. The interplay between psychiatry and political expedience was to characterize the early months of that year.

The issue of the alleged apology made by the United States to Canada continued to occupy center stage. During the winter of 1986, the Canadian Justice Department sent two representatives to Washington to evaluate the materials held by the CIA. Initially, these men refused to meet with our lawyers, Joe Rauh and Jim Turner. They did finally agree to a briefing but did not review at length the material that had been prepared for the court. Ultimately their work was to assist significantly the defense of the CIA.

Rauh and Turner were now fighting against an opponent who held all the cards. They were not permitted to obtain any more documents from the CIA. The two agency men who were said to have tendered the apology were not permitted to testify. Thus began a series of letters between these attorneys and senior Canadian government representatives. The onus was on the Canadian government; if it said that an apology had been offered, it should either release any appropriate documentation, or make available for testimony John Hadwen, the former liaison officer who was said to have received the statement of "regret." If Hadwen testified about the substance of the apology, as well as who had given it, the CIA would then have to allow Knaus and Hulse, the former CIA station agents in Ottawa, to testify as well. The ball was in the Canadians' court.

In late January, the attorneys received an affidavit from Hadwen; although a legal document, it was inadmissible in an American court because Hadwen would not be subject to cross-examination. In sum, it was a useless contribution. Its contents, however, were promising. As reported by the *Ottawa Citizen* on February 13, 1986:

> The statement says that Hadwen called in U.S. embassy representatives in September, 1977 to complain about the CIA-funded MKULTRA project, ". . . protesting not only the failure to consult, but the nature of the programme."
>
> "I know that the official sent to meet with me expressed regret," Hadwen's statement says, "His regret certainly ap-

> plied to CIA funding of the research in Montreal without our knowledge, but I also believe he expressed regret at the nature of the programme."

Again, Rauh and Turner made representations to Canada. If Clark truly wished to help these Canadian citizens, Hadwen had to be deposed with attorneys of both sides present. On Monday, February 10, 1986, Clark turned down the request. The *Citizen* article goes on:

> A government source close to the case said another reason [in addition to Clark's contention that the affidavit was sufficient] Ottawa was leery of sending Hadwen to testify was that Rauh could start probing the sensitive intelligence relationship between the United States and Canada.

From the beginning, the CIA had stated that Canada was more responsible for the funding of Cameron's work, that its own contribution had been minor. The request regarding Hadwen was an opportunity for the Canadian government to attack the credibility of this assertion. It was difficult to understand Clark's reasoning and his decision.

Two days later, Canada's Prime Minister Mulroney undercut his external affairs minister, clearing the way for Hadwen to be deposed. It is painful to consider what then transpired. At the deposition, which took place in Ottawa, Hadwen was prevented by the representatives of the External Affairs and Justice Departments from providing other than basic information. The lawyers from Canada joined with the CIA attorneys to prevent Hadwen from naming the CIA official who had proffered the apology. The Canadian attitude during the deposition became increasingly hostile, and Hadwen was left to respond to questions by reading the public statements of the current and former external affairs ministers. He was advised not to answer any questions involving the CIA.

How can one understand this ambivalent response by the Canadian government? Did they in fact have something to hide about their own involvement? Did issues of thirty years ago so imperil intelligence concerns that they would abandon the defense of their own citizens? The worst was yet to come.

During the summer of 1985, Minister of Justice John Crosbie had asked for what has been termed an independent opinion of the work at the Allan Memorial, and Canada's involvement in this work. He commissioned George Cooper, a Halifax attorney, former Conservative member of Parliament, and law partner of a current cabinet minister, to carry out the investigation. Mr. Cooper summarizes his instructions as follows:

> You have asked for my opinion on certain matters related to activities carried on at the Allan Memorial Institute ("AMI") in Montreal during the 1950s and 1960s by Dr. D. Ewen Cameron and others, and in particular as to whether in the funding of these activities the Government of Canada did anything or omitted to do anything which might be found to be illegal or improper if an action were brought or a complaint made by one or more former patients at the AMI.

Cooper's reference to Canada's support of Cameron's work is significant. The Cooper Report, issued in May 1986, is pivotal to an understanding of subsequent events because it lays out in significant detail a model for how both the Canadian and American governments could escape responsibility for funding a research project that led to such a tragic outcome. The report was damaging to the search for truth in several ways. First, it provided a basis for the Canadian government to wash its hands of involvement; second, it supported what several Canadian psychiatrists had claimed—that Cameron's work was standard in its time; third, it gave all the ammunition to the CIA that it required to file for dismissal of the case; and last, the report offered legal and ethical arguments against governmental and individual responsibility for the research.

After I read the report, I was outraged. The data gathered reflected a poor attempt to be comprehensive; no questions were asked of the patients, their families, or the attorneys.

Consequently, Cooper's interpretation of the data was wide open and highly questionable.

The first section of the report examines the psychiatric procedures that were used at the Allan Memorial Institute during the years from 1948 through 1964. Cooper divided these into two main categories: procedures used elsewhere in Canada and the world, including ECT, insulin comas, sleep therapy, and drugs (including LSD); and a second group, which were procedures used at the Allan and at a few centers in some other countries (but not elsewhere in Canada). Within this group, he included depatterning, psychic driving, and sensory isolation. His conclusion was that "none of the foregoing psychiatric procedures were pioneered at the Allan, and none were unique to it. . . ." This is nonsense. Depatterning with shock treatment was prescribed elsewhere for last-stage schizophrenic or other severely disturbed patients for whom nothing else had worked. But no one had used all of Cameron's combinations to depattern. I have been unable to find any other center in the world where psychic driving and sensory isolation were used to treat patients.

In trying to explain Cameron's theoretical framework, Cooper notes the theory behind depatterning and states that "Dr. Cameron took hold of this idea and developed it further than psychiatrists in the mainstream of European and North American practice." He suggests that the theory that formed the basis for psychic driving was based on the idea of "remothering" in a procedure called "anaclitic therapy." This "remothering" procedure, which had been pioneered at the Allan by Hassan Azima, utilized sensory isolation to foster a significant amount of regression and dependency in patients. Their enormous needs were then met through the therapist's spending inordinate amounts of time taking care of their basic requirements and, in a sense, duplicating and improving upon their early mothering, which may have been problematic or disturbed. Although one may question Azima's approach, it was humane, and patients could leave at any time. Cameron's work, on the other hand, did not involve "remothering" in any form; the repetition of messages from a disembodied voice can hardly be described as a nurturing process. Cooper's comparison of the theory behind psychic driving with the nurturing "remothering" treatment simply does not wash.

Cooper suggests that, in the selection of patients, Cameron concentrated on schizophrenic or long term chronic psychoneurotic people for whom all prior types of treatment had failed. Yet we know that Cameron's application of psychotherapeutic treatment likely did not extend beyond a cursory attempt. Indeed, since he did not believe in classical psychotherapy and felt it to be too slow, he was apt to abandon it rather hastily and move on to his preferred intrusive treatments.

From data gathered for John Marks's book, and documents in the archives of the American Psychiatric Association, it is apparent that some of Cameron's patients were kept in isolation far longer than the sixteen days that Cooper has cited. However, even more relevant is the fact that, before Cameron, researchers had used only volunteer subjects in sensory deprivation experimentation, and their maximum reported stay had been five to six days. It is incorrect to compare Cameron's "depatterning" with that conducted by other groups for three reasons; first, no one used the combinations of techniques Cameron did; second, patient selection was not comparable; third, other groups saw depatterning as last-stage treatment only.

Cooper suggests that Cameron's use of drugs was no different from that of other Canadian psychiatrists in the 1950s and 1960s. Once again, this is an overstatement. Certainly LSD, amphetamines, and barbiturates had been tried in many centers. But no one combined these drugs with such ferocity, and experimental drugs such as PCP (Sernyl) were not routinely used.

Cooper concludes that, with respect to theory and treatment, these procedures "were not based on sound principles of science and medicine" and that depatterning "represented a level of assault on the brain that was not justifiable even by the standards of the time and even in light of the rather rudimentary level of scientific and medical knowledge of those days compared to today." He goes on to remark that no doctors spoke out at the time, and in fact, none at the time of Cooper's report were willing to attribute improper motivations to Cameron. Thus, despite all the justification for Cameron's practices, Cooper concludes with a critical analysis of the work. It appears somehow odd that Cooper is unable to state clearly that the work was unacceptable. I can only explain this by concluding that Cooper's principal purpose in writing the report was to protect the Canadian government. Ultimately, of course, the medical profession rejected all of Cameron's work in this area; it was never used elsewhere at McGill or anywhere in the world—perhaps this is the most significant statement of all.

After assessing Cameron's work, the Cooper Report went on to examine how Cameron obtained funding. Cooper revealed that the Government of Canada had, in fact, provided significant funds for Cameron's research during the 1950s. The Defence Research Board of Canada funded one project that was likely related to sensory isolation work—namely, a study of "Behavioural Problems in the Adaptation of White Man to the Arctic." The Canadian Department of Health and Welfare provided three grants: the first, Project No. 604-5-14 (1950–54), provided Can. $17,875 to a "Behavioural Laboratory"; experiments there included work with intensive shock treatment, sensory isolation, and psychic driving. The second grant, Project No. 604-5-432 (1961–64), provided Can. $51,860 for a project entitled "Study of Factors which Promote or Retard Personality Change in Individuals Exposed to Prolonged Repetition of Verbal Signals"—in other words, psychic driving. A third grant was dismissed by Cooper as irrelevant. This was Project No. 604-5-74 (1959–61), titled "A Study of Ultraconceptual Communication," which was conducted under the direction of Leonard Rubenstein. How this project could be irrelevant puzzles me since Cameron and Rubenstein described it as being based on a study of the process of driving. They noted that "constant repetition, particularly as far as the patient is concerned[,] may result in an exhaustion of his defences." Ultraconceptual communication thus referred to the process of sending signals that are beyond the level of awareness. The work represented a new dimension in the process of mind control.

Cooper assesses the mechanism by which grant applications were reviewed in Canada at that time. He indicates that Cameron's applications received no special consideration, but he also suggests that "it is likely that some readers of the reviewing groups may have been somewhat reluctant to express doubts. . . ." Indeed, "in the view of many of them [people who participated in review], Dr. Cameron's preeminence in the field, added to his forceful and aggressive personality, may well have resulted in a certain deference being shown to his applications. . . ." Despite these reservations, Mr. Cooper states that there is no evidence that the Canadian Department of Health and Welfare did anything imprudent with respect to Cameron's applications.

The report then turns to the highly controversial and enigmatic D. Ewen Cameron. Clearly, Cooper has some difficulty in reconciling the extreme intrusiveness of Cameron's physical methods of treatment with his own perspective of psychiatry as a humane science. He tries to explain away any criticisms of Cameron's work in the following way. Cooper notes correctly that there existed two schools of psychiatry at the time—the psychoanalytic and the "physical" school; Cameron belonged, as we know, to the latter. But Cooper is totally incorrect when he says: "The fact that in the years since 1964 the physical approach has fallen out of fashion in favour of the analytical approach, makes it more difficult for psychiatrists and others to look at the problem through 1950s and 1960s eyes (as we must in passing judgment both legal and ethical) rather than through the eyes of the 1980s."

This is absurd. The principal change that psychiatry has undergone as a profession has been the recognition of the biological nature of many psychiatric illnesses. The growth of psychopharmacology, and newer diagnostic technologies such as positron emission tomography, all suggest that biological psychiatry is alive and well. Indeed, the chairmanships of most major departments of psychiatry in the United States moved during those years from pure analysts to biologists or biologists who had also been analytically trained. The major advances in our understanding of human behavior have in recent times grown out of research in biochemistry and neurophysiology. Cooper's argument is therefore spurious.

Not surprisingly, Cooper acknowledges that Cameron was a poor scientist. He especially points out the inadequacy of his work with respect to assessment of efficacy. He reports Cameron's ignorance of the placebo effect of increased attention from staff, or from being inside a hospital, or from being placed on a new drug. The report explains this away by pointing out that there was a dearth of psychiatrists in the 1950s; psychiatry was a young science with a definite lack of knowledge and a crying need for research. Cooper then gathers evidence from other psychiatrists, especially Cameron's successor, Cleghorn, that the work was not any less rigorous than that carried out by others at the time. He quotes Cleghorn: "It was the 20 to 25 year period from 1935 (i.e., 1955 to 1960) before the concept of adequate controls (such as making allowances for the Hawthorne and placebo effects) had assumed a regular place in medical research, *and longer for psychiatry, for it had less involvement than medicine in the basic sciences, therefore was even more laggardly* [emphasis added]." What the report does not consider is the vast improvement in research methodology that took place from the late 1950s onward when Cameron's research was evolving. It is true that the work was published; it is also true that it was never taken up or replicated by other researchers. Perhaps because it was not respected?

Cooper does note that several psychologists with whom he spoke were more skeptical than the medical doctors. He comments that they were more scientifically trained and thus more capable of critical examination. Yet the premise that more rigorous research methodology was not being employed by other psychiatrists deserves examination. Consider a paper written by a member of Cameron's department, Heinz Lehmann. It was published in 1960, which means that it was written in 1958–59; it is therefore based on the thinking of the late 1950s—the very time when Cameron's work was being carried out. The title of the piece is "The Place and Purpose of Objective Methods in Psychopharmacology," and it appears in a book that is titled *Drugs and Behavior.*

Lehmann alludes to the "ever increasing use of objective methods in . . . research, and the need for a systematic approach to research." This, he suggests, "implies, in addition to the gathering of observational data, their rational analysis, an elimination of subjective bias, and finally, the construction and testing of hypotheses and theories." He raises questions of reliability, validity, and objectivity in research and assesses the relative weights of nine different methods with respect to these issues. For example, he suggests that physiological tests are the most objective, and observation by others the least reliable. He raises the issue of "placebo response" and describes a study of his that used a "double-blind methodology." The issue of control groups is also considered.

What all of this scientific terminology means is that in order for researchers to ascertain whether a treatment or other intervention works, they must use a set of procedures that will ensure that the results make sense and are reliable. For example, if patients in a hospital are placed on a new drug, how can we know that the drug makes a difference? It might be that the giving of a new pill alone will produce change—this is "placebo response." If one group of patients were given the medication and a similar group were given a pill without medication, then perhaps we would have a better sense of whether the medication is effective. Similarly, if the researchers know which patients are receiving the medication, they might somehow treat them differently; thus a good research design hides, both from the subjects and from the experimenters, the information on who is receiving the drug. This is known as a "double-blind" study.

Lehmann was not the only psychiatrist considering these issues. In September 1956, the National Institute of Mental Health, the National Academy of Sciences–National Research Council, and the American Psychiatric Association sponsored a conference on "The Evaluation of Pharmacotherapy in Mental Illness." The proceedings were published in a book entitled *Psychopharmacology: Problems in Eval-*

uation. The range of topics was broad. Ralph Gerard, one of the editors, raised several issues that must be considered in "sound clinical investigation": these included "the selection of the experimental and control populations, the testing conditions, the criteria for evaluating change, the follow-up procedures, the quantitative judgments, and the proprieties of reporting results." Controlled studies that use statistical methods to evaluate the use of chlorpromazine and reserpine were presented in a paper by Evarts and Butler. Louis Lasagna (who was to make significant contributions to psychopharmacology) and Victor Laties reviewed problems in the study of drugs such as drug dosage, mode and timing of administration, sampling and individual differences, experimental procedures, and use of controls. They comment: "Placebo and double-blind controls are of proven value in experimental work, and the reasons for their use should not need to be discussed at length in the year 1956." The conference addressed multiple issues in clinical research—from halo effects to randomization of clinical subjects. Once again, these are scientific terms that refer to research-design issues that must be considered to ensure that results are valid.

This meeting, which occurred in the same year that Cameron published his paper on "Psychic Driving," represented the state of the art in psychiatry at that time. To say, therefore, that Cameron's shoddy research design was typical of that produced by psychiatry in the mid-1950s is simply untrue. As chairman of a major department, as well as a past president of the American Psychiatric Association, Cameron was surely aware of the meeting. The fact that his own work did not reflect the thinking of researchers in the "physical" aspects of psychiatry suggests that Cameron chose either to ignore contemporary experimental standards and methods or did not have the patience or expertise to carry out acceptable research.

Some have excused Cameron on the basis that his work was not in fact experimentation at all—it was merely an extension of treatment. Available evidence does not support this view. Experimentation involves the development of a series of procedures designed to test a theory. The purpose of the procedures is to generate knowledge that may or may not benefit the subject of the experiment. The individual's needs are less important than discovering something about the pathology of the illness or the treatment of a disease. Cameron's work did not constitute standard treatment, and grant monies were obtained to build a behavioral laboratory. Both Cameron and his associate referred to their work as experiments. There is no question, then, that Ewen Cameron was acting in the capacity of a research investigator with respect to this work.

It is sad that Lehmann's concluding remarks in his paper could not have been applied at that time to Ewen Cameron:

> I should like to conclude my discussion with a plea that the development of objective evaluation standards for a clinical psychiatrist's performance be seriously considered, not necessarily with regard to his success as a therapist, but with respect to his competence as a diagnostician, a prognostician, and a research worker. One could conceive of methods that would permit "calibration" of the performance of a clinical research-psychiatrist in a manner similar to the calibration of a complex research instrument. . . . His sensitivity, bias, recording ability, and stability of performance should be used to better advantage as a research instrument than is now being done.

Cooper's conclusion that Cameron was a "good doctor" but was a poor researcher makes no sense. A good doctor does not ignore the work being done in his field and thereby place his patients at risk. Cooper also notes that "this was not a case of 'experiments' carried out on socially disadvantaged patients who were under compulsion or did not know any better." They were voluntary, says he. Yes, voluntary patients; they did not volunteer to be subjects in research experiments. To follow his reasoning, one has to ask: Is it a comfort, after you have paid thousands of dollars and lost all of your money, to know that you had the privilege of having been experimented upon?

The rest of Cooper's discussion of Cameron's work in the context of the time is filled with contradictions. At times hearsay evidence, such as the opinions of the psychologists, is ignored; at other times, it is accepted. We are given the opinion of Cleghorn, who "knows personally of no patient of whom it could be said with *certainty* that they were worse off because of the depatterning procedures than they otherwise would have been [emphasis in the original]." This flies in the face of the demonstration of organic brain damage in the follow-up study on the effects of depatterning carried out by Schwartzman and Termansen.

It is interesting that Cooper relied upon the opinions of three experts in the field of psychiatry. Quotes from their reports raise interesting questions. Professor Frederic Grunberg, Department of Psychiatry, University of Montreal, notes: "I personally disagree and disagreed then with the intrusiveness and lack of scientific rigor of his work." His conclusion: "There is no evidence that psychic driving did any irreparable harm to patients who voluntary [*sic*] submitted to it. The Canadian Government should not bare [*sic*] any moral responsibility for supporting a project that was essentially therapeutic in its aims."

Dean Ian McDonald of the University of Saskatchewan writes with respect to Cameron's attempts to reduce disability in schizophrenics: "His method of achieving this, however, I think is seriously open to question because of the use of two techniques which carried a not inconsiderable risk and which hitherto had not been established as being effective."

Frederick Lowy, then Dean of Medicine at the University of Toronto, writes:

> There were many skeptics, even in his department at McGill. Many psychiatrists in Canada and abroad considered the treatment methods extreme, overly risky and/or without proper theoretical foundation. . . . his criteria for the selection of patients for these controversial treatments seemed to broaden. By the time I became personally involved with his patients (1961) it was my own view that many of the schizophrenic patients who were "depatterned" had not had adequate trials of appropriate phenothiazine medications that were then available and many of the psychoneurotic patients who received hallucinogenic drugs and psychic driving could have been helped by conventional psychotherapy. Of course, at the

> time I was very junior in status and quite inexperienced in psychiatry; nevertheless, even in hindsight after more than twenty years of practicing and teaching psychiatry I still hold this view.

Two of the three experts, then, disagreed with Cameron *at the time*, while the third wonders at the intrusiveness and experimental nature of the "treatment." Yet Cooper concludes that "the Government of Canada cannot be expected to bear responsibility for what happened at the AMI, even assuming (contrary to my own conclusion on the point) that Dr. Cameron crossed over the line of the acceptable in medical research."

In one of the most startling aspects of the Cooper Report, Cooper then devotes nineteen pages to a discussion of the role of the CIA in funding the work of Ewen Cameron. This is puzzling, since it would appear to exceed the instruction that he was given. In any event, this part of the report is a poorly crafted defense of the CIA's position. It does not draw upon material from Rauh and Turner that would have painted quite a different picture.

Cooper's conclusion (which is the contention of the CIA) is that "the CIA was only involved in funding and was not involved in instigating, directing and controlling Cameron's work; and that Cameron was simply applying treatments of a kind which . . . had become standard practice for him." Thus, not only is the Canadian government relieved of any responsibility, but the American government becomes absolved as well. He then acknowledges the funding by the Society for the Investigation of Human Ecology, but states that the CIA-funded work merely built on what had gone before. Clearly, the grant application and papers published during the funding period indicate that Cameron was planning to become even more aggressive in his approaches to the breaking down of defenses and in the sophistication of the reprogramming method of psychic driving. The question of whether the "treatments" were solely for the benefit of the patients or "pure experiments" is cavalierly dismissed by such statements as "all of the medical people with whom I spoke were strongly inclined to doubt it, as were almost all the others I spoke to." In this instance, opinions and hearsay become conclusive evidence.

Cooper then presents some considerations that can only represent great naiveté. He wonders how a CIA agent could keep his purposes and affiliation secret from colleagues and staff. More than one hundred researchers of MKULTRA did just that; in fact, the CIA was able to convince the United States Supreme Court that these names should never be revealed. He goes on to comment on Cameron's published works and lectures, and concludes: "It seems to me a servant of the CIA would have kept a lower profile." Indeed, many of those who have been publicly identified as CIA MKULTRA researchers, such as Harold Abramson, Harold Wolff, Robert Hyde, and Harris Isbell, have published their research results widely.

Cooper ignores the deposition of John Gittinger in which he acknowledges that the Society approached Cameron and solicited his application. Instead, he relies on an earlier deposition (1977) that would rule out Cameron's complicity. Cooper then suggests that even if Cameron did know that the money came from the CIA, this did not necessarily mean ill intent. "Like many scientists," he posits, "Cameron would take grant money wherever he could without taint." Yet many scientists did not; John Marks describes how John Lilly, who was working at the National Institutes of Health on brain mapping and sensory isolation, had "officials of the CIA and other agencies descend upon him with a request for a briefing." He agreed "only under the condition that it and his work remain unclassified, completely open to outsiders." He goes on to state: "Lilly realized that the intelligence agencies were not interested in sensory deprivation because of its positive benefits, and he finally concluded that it was impossible for him to work at the National Institutes of Health without compromising his principles. He quit in 1958." Some scientists are men of honor.

There is another piece of data that sheds light on the role of the CIA in mind-control research. At the time of taking the deposition of Admiral Stansfield Turner, the former Director of Central Intelligence, Rauh and Turner requested to see the manuscript of Turner's then forthcoming book

Secrecy and Democracy. Although there was some reluctance on Turner's part to comply with this request, the attorneys were allowed to hear a dictated description of the relevant text on MKULTRA. The paragraph went as follows:

> How could this [MKULTRA] have happened? I believe compartmentation was responsible. Because of compartmentation there was inadequate supervision of those who, with good intent, concocted this absurd scheme. The unit conducting the experiment simply had such autonomy that not many outsiders could look in and ask what was going on. In all walks of life people get too close to their work and need someone with a somewhat detached viewpoint to take an occasional look at where they are going. In this case the system just could not provide that kind of detached critical review and a few well-intentioned but terribly misguided individuals badly abused the CIA's privilege of keeping secret so much of what it does.

This paragraph would appear to be an admission of negligence. It, and many other passages, were excised from the book at the insistence of the CIA.

Yet, despite all of this, Cooper presents a defense of the CIA, terming the question of their involvement, a "red herring." It is interesting that Cooper acknowledges in the report the assistance of M. L. Jewett, Q.C., General Counsel, Constitutional and International Law, of the Canadian Justice Department, and Louis B. Z. Davis of the same section of the department. These were the men who visited Washington at the beginning of the year, and who spent a significant amount of time with the CIA and little time with Rauh and Turner. Within one week of publication of the Cooper Report, the CIA was citing this section as Canada's support of its position of innocence.

Although the report includes a section on the ethical considerations that surround Cameron's research, including the issue of informed consent, Cooper gives only a rather cursory glance at these issues—issues that many feel are major reasons Cameron's work should have been rejected when it first took place. Cooper does examine some of the precedents that bear on this critical aspect of the case, but those that he cites tend to date from after 1964. Strikingly absent is any mention of the Nuremberg Code of medical ethics. There is a wealth of literature, both legal and historical, that relates to ethical considerations in scientific research. It is surprising that the report did not examine this literature in much greater detail.

Following the section on ethics, Cooper turns to the legal principles that he felt were applicable in this case. After an examination of several of these principles, he concludes that "the Crown is not legally liable for the conduct of Dr. Cameron. . . ." As to the question of propriety of the treatments, he notes: "Perhaps the conclusion that comes closest to the truth is that he acted incautiously, but not irresponsibly. . . ." His final opinion: "Given the climate of the times, and the prevailing practices as to medical research and experimentation, ethics and consent, the Government of Canada cannot be expected to bear responsibility for what happened at the AMI. . . . It is difficult to see how moral responsibility can lie on the government in such a situation. . . ." His final conclusion falls back on a principle that clouded malpractice law for many years—the notion that a doctor must have the latitude to make mistakes.

The response of the media to the Cooper Report was immediate. The *Montreal Gazette*, in an editorial on May 9, 1986, noted that "nothing can absolve Ottawa of its moral responsibility toward the victims." The *Ottawa Citizen* on the same day said, "John Crosbie was right to commission, and release, the lawyer's opinion on the government's role in the so-called CIA brainwashing case. He was wrong to adopt that opinion. . . ." It noted that Cooper provided an excuse for Cameron's conduct by saying that "it is wrong to apply present-day ethical standards to actions of a different era." It then declared that this excuse "crumbles under the weight of precedents. We apply fresh moral insight all the time to past behaviour; the government is doing that now as it considers compensation to Japanese-Canadians for wartime dispossessions." In a letter to the *Toronto Globe and Mail*, I wrote, "And so the tragedy continues. Aided and abetted by the Government of Canada, promoted by the lack of response of the medical profession, eight Canadians see their lives amount to nothing. . . . Are there any Canadians who care?" By this time, one of the original plaintiffs had passed away.

My letter was prompted by what I saw as a total lack of compassion and a sense of responsibility on the part of the Government of Canada. Other than Ed Broadbent, then leader of the New Democratic Party, of which David Orlikow was an old and respected member, and Svend Robinson, another NDP member, not one member of Parliament either raised questions in the House or otherwise demonstrated that this issue was of any importance. Yet this was an issue of Canadian sovereignty. An American government agency had stepped in and funded research on Canadian citizens as part of an extensive program of mind control experimentation. It was certainly apparent to me that if the shoe had been on the other foot, the ruckus in Congress would have reached heretofore unheard-of heights. I was stunned by the silence and began to ask myself what Canada was all about? Was it merely a satellite of its giant neighbor?

When I was growing up in Montreal, there was a sense that anything American was better. People used to drive from Montreal and its fine shops to Burlington, Vermont, or Plattsburgh, New York, to shop for what were often inferior clothes or trinkets. The girls wanted American boyfriends, and American television was better. There are two implications to all of this. First, it is exceedingly difficult to maintain a national identity in a country where twenty-five million people are strung along a three-thousand–mile band of territory that lies within two hundred miles of the American border. Second, the concept of the longest undefended border also allows for significant American input at all levels—input that threatens the development of distinctive Canadian culture. In an editorial quoted in a Dartmouth College report on Canadian-American relations, the *Montreal Star* on January 7, 1967, stated:

> No one can live on this continent, or even on this planet, without being aware of the saturating force of American civ-

> ilization. We begin then, with the proposition that in dealing with the United States, we are dealing with something not necessarily bad but which exists, with what Toynbee has called the American empire, a form of economic and cultural imperialism. . . . The Alternative Is To Be Ourselves: We are a country; we have our interests and policies; we should conduct them on the basis of knowing what we want to achieve.

Canadians have not clarified their goals as a people. Several authors have pointed out that searching for a Canadian identity is a national pastime. As John Holmes says, "Sovereignty is something Canadians may worry about, but they agonize about their identity." Peter Desbarats, in his book *Canada Lost/Canada Found: The Search for a New Nation*, decries Canada's rejection of its proud past; he sees Canadians as promulgating myths of their own inadequacies, of how they "drifted into nationhood." He says: "We are a nation that has lost its sense of history. We don't even understand that we have not always been as we are today, ignorant and confused about our past, uncertain about ourselves, and skeptical about the future." We are thus left with a country that puts itself down, and that struggles to maintain unity in a federal system of government that allows provinces great independence. Given this framework, relations with the United States become problematic.

In the United States, as Canadians know only too well, Canada is very much taken for granted. Virtually no Canadian news is found on radio, television, or in the newspapers of the United States. Knowledge of Canadian geography, government, or economics is extremely limited. There are moments when Canada is acknowledged to exist, such as when the Canadian Embassy in Iran saved the lives of American hostages, or when Americans suddenly realize how much real estate in the United States is owned by Canadians. But for the most part, Canada is perceived only as the place where the cold weather fronts arise. Holmes asks whether Americans have progressed

> . . . in their approach to a country which, the facts of geography and economics suggest, ought to be of primary im-

> portance. The political leaders continue to treat us as a child nation, to be humored with fraternal speeches while our specific complaints are pooh-poohed away. The fact that President Carter visited almost every capital except Ottawa is itself less infuriating than the bland American explanation so often offered—that there are not enough problems between us to warrant a visit. There is something refreshing about the concentrated hostility of the *Wall Street Journal*. They do take us seriously, while President Reagan invokes the memory of Mary Pickford to exorcise any differences such fine folks might have.

Many authors have explored two aspects of Canadian culture that offer an explanation, both for the ambivalent assistance that the Canadian government has offered and for the dearth of response from the Canadian public. David Baldwin, in a 1967 discussion of Canadian-American relations, notes that the Canadian approach to international affairs over the years has been, "Don't rock the boat. Things will turn out fine if you leave everything to behind-the-scenes diplomacy." Holmes says,

> It is important to our material well-being that we be regarded by Congress and the administration as a good ally, although we should never allow ourselves to be blackmailed or bought. . . . our first priority should be the seeking of compromise, that old smoothie role so much deplored in recent years.

Elsewhere, he remarks that "Canadians suffer more often from the delusion that human wrongs in other countries can be righted by a strong speech or stiff note from the Canadian ambassador." Canada, therefore, has always opted for quiet diplomacy. Yet, as Baldwin again points out:

> Quiet diplomacy is not always more effective than squeaky wheel diplomacy. In a discussion of peaceful settlement of disputes, Iris Claude ruefully admits that "states are likely to get what they want if they raise sufficient fuss, and unlikely to get it if they fail to do so."

Baldwin's pithy solution—"The quickest way for Canada to

get the United States to stop taking it for granted is to make trouble." But that is not the Canadian way.

The second cultural attribute has been well described by June Callwood and Peter Desbarats. Callwood describes the ready acceptance by Canadians of the virtual suspension of civil liberties by the War Measures Act of 1970, whereby Prime Minister Trudeau was given significant powers to curb the sporadic terrorist bombings in the province of Quebec. She writes:

> Canadians tolerate even brutal use of authority without disapproval. Unless it is directed at them personally, they don't mind. They trust the government and police to act in the best interests of society even when they do not seem to be doing so. They trust that authority knows best. . . . Canada developed from people who consciously, and with some considerable sacrifice, chose structure rather than individualism and wanted a powerful state rather than citizen rights. While the American constitution speaks of liberty, the Canadian one says "peace, order, and good government."

Desbarats also comments on this apparent blind acceptance of state authority. He describes the absence of a sense of outrage by Canadians in response to the revelations that the Royal Canadian Mounted Police had been opening mail; committing arson, theft, and illegal surveillance; and providing misleading information to the cabinet. He writes: "Moral outrage in public affairs doesn't exist in Canada except as a hackneyed device in political speeches, and this is accepted as a conventional exercise in futility by everyone."

Another point Desbarats makes is that senior civil servants, rather than elected officials, make and control public policy. He says, "In Canada, bureaucratic values now attempt to shape our national structure." Can it be that bureaucratic values have shaped the response of the Canadian government to the CIA in the Cameron case? Did these same values influence the thrust of the Cooper opinion? Am I just experiencing, at first hand, a combination of Canadian apathy and of a government approach to the United States that emphasizes the advantage of not making waves? If so, one must ask whether Canada as a country truly stands up for its own sovereignty, whether it is capable as a nation of defending the rights of its citizens. Cooper suggests that the Canadian government has no legal or moral responsibility for what happened to nine Canadians. The legalities are open to debate, but all democratic governments have a moral responsibility to their citizenry, in this situation no less than any other.

And so, psychiatry and politics have been enmeshed in this case for more than thirty years. The relationship has taken many turns. Today the emphasis is on international diplomacy. The complex involvement of the United States and Canada thus becomes the focus either for resolution of the Cameron case, or for the sacrifice of Cameron's victims on the altar of political expediency.

There remained one further area that I needed to explore. What was there to be learned in the history of medicine and human experimentation?

In many ways, this facet of understanding has remained one of the most difficult aspects of the case. Since I am a physician, and because I feel so deeply the obligation of my profession to care for human life, the concept of experimentation on unknowing individuals is one that evokes great feelings of revulsion. Yet human experimentation has been a necessary component of research into the causes of disease. Weighing the rights of patients against the desire to achieve understanding and the ability to cure human illness requires a balanced and judicious interpretation of the limits of experimental research. Consequently, achieving this balance has occupied the profession over many years. Medicine alone has not made these determinations, for it is the law, as it protects the rights of patients and the prerogatives of physicians, that ultimately defines what is acceptable. It was important, then, to understand how Ewen Cameron's work was outside the realm of what was acceptable—not only within medicine, but within the law as well.

15

Medical Ethics and Human Experimentation: Nuremberg, Montreal, and Now

I will use treatment to help the sick according to my ability and judgment, but never with a view to injury and wrong-doing. Neither will I administer a poison to anybody. . . .

—*Hippocratic Oath*

Experiments, then may be performed on man, but within what limits? It is our duty and our right to perform an experiment on man whenever it can save his life, cure him or gain him some personal benefit. The principle of medical and surgical morality, therefore, consists in never performing on man an experiment which might be harmful to him to any extent, even though the result might be highly advantageous to science, i.e. to the health of others. . . .

—*Claude Bernard, 1865*

> Under no circumstances is a doctor permitted to do anything that would weaken the physical or mental resistance of a human being except from strictly professional reasons in the interest of his patient. . . . A doctor is advised to use good caution in publishing discoveries. The same applies to methods of treatment whose value is not recognized by the profession.
>
> —*World Medical Association, Declaration of Geneva, 1948, under "Duties of Doctors in General"*

Medicine has a long tradition of following a set of ideals that hold the human body to be a sacred vessel; the physician-priest is admonished to handle the vessel with care and reverence. The dictum *primum non nocere*—above all, do no harm—has been the byword of the profession for centuries. The importance of ethical behavior in medicine has been emphasized many times. In earlier years, ethical precepts have focused upon the behavior of physicians toward each other, but in this century ethical standards have come increasingly to focus upon decision making in medical care. Recent concerns have focused upon abortion, genetic counseling, the high costs and limits of technology, and the maintenance of life by machines in the face of irreversible coma. The ethical issues that confront medicine are complex and force physicians to examine daily their values and beliefs; unfortunately, few medical schools adequately prepare their students for this task.

In 1946–47, twenty-three physicians stood in the dock at Nuremberg accused of perpetrating the most heinous crimes against humanity in the name of science. As Brigadier General Taylor noted:

> [They] . . . range from leaders of German scientific medicine, with excellent international scientific reputations, down to the dregs of the German medical profession. All of them have in common a callous lack of consideration and human regard for, and an unprincipled willingness to abuse their power, over the poor, unfortunate, defenseless creatures who had been deprived of their rights by a ruthless and criminal gov-

> ernment. All of them violated the Hippocratic commandments which they had solemnly sworn to uphold and abide by. . . .

Part of the physicians' defense was that human experimentation had been occurring in the world for many years; in fact, drawing upon world literature, they were able to point to experiments that involved more than eleven thousand people. In other words, it was acceptable to carry out this kind of research because it was being done elsewhere. Dr. Robert Servatius, counsel for one of the defendants, noted in his final plea,

> It is repeatedly shown that the experiments for which no consent was given were permitted with the full knowledge of the government authorities. It is further shown that these experiments were published in professional literature without meeting any objection, and that they were even accepted by the public without concern as a natural phenomenon when reports about them appeared in popular magazines.

This defense was not acceptable to the tribunal, partly because of the testimony of Dr. Andrew C. Ivy of the United States. Ivy stated that, as far as he knew, no deaths had occurred in these experiments, except in one case where the experimenters had used themselves as experimental subjects and two had died. With respect to the issue of consent by subjects to experimentation, Ivy was questioned about the standards adopted by the American Medical Association in 1946. The testimony went as follows:

> Q. What was the basis on which the American Medical Association adopted these rules?
>
> A. I submitted to them a report of certain experiments which had been performed on human subjects along with my conclusions as to what the principles of ethics should be for use of human beings in medical experiments. . . .
>
> Q. Well now, you have, first of all, a basic requirement for experimentation on human beings . . . [that is] . . . the voluntary consent of the individual upon whom the experiment is to be performed must be obtained.

> A. Yes.
>
> Q. Now does that purport to be the principles upon which all physicians and scientists guide themselves before they resort to medical experimentation on human beings in the United States?
>
> A. Yes. They represent the basic principles approved by the American Medical Association for the use of human beings as subjects in medical experiments.
>
> Judge Sebring: How do the principles which you have just enunciated comport with the principles of the medical profession over the civilized world generally?
>
> A. They are identical, according to my information. . . .

Ivy, in a paper describing his testimony at Nuremberg, notes the other two principles that characterized experimentation in American medicine during the war. These included, first, the need to base the experiment upon the results of animal research and upon knowledge of the natural course of the disease that was the focus of study; second, it was essential that the work be carried out by qualified investigators. He added: "In other words, whenever there has been danger attached to any experiment, any *a priori* hazard, it has been honorable medically for the experimenters also to serve as subjects."

It is chilling and almost unbearable to contemporary physicians to consider the number of physicians who were involved in the Nazi experimentation. M. H. Pappworth notes that over two hundred doctors were named, including "many professors of medicine and others in official positions of power in the medical hierarchy of the Third Reich." He quotes Ivy in suggesting that hundreds more were aware of the work. Pappworth continues:

> 'The cooperation and active participation of all these doctors was spontaneous when they realized that the opportunity to experiment on humans far beyond normal limits was presented to them. Not one of the convicted doctors ever acknowledged that they had done anything wrong whatsoever or expressed the slightest remorse.

A prosecution witness at Nuremberg, Professor Werner Leibrandt, suggested that the Nazi doctors labored under a phenomenon called biological thought. He explained:

> By biological thought I mean the attitude of a physician who does not take the subject into consideration at all, but for whom the patient has become a mere object, so that the human relationship no longer exists, and a man becomes a mere object like a small package.

Professor Michael Kater of York University, Toronto, has noted that almost 45% of German physicians joined the Nazi Party. Even more frightening, he describes how, following the war, the German medical establishment rewarded and promoted ex-Nazi physicians so that they came to hold many of the valued teaching positions in the medical faculties of the universities.

Out of the judgment of the military tribunal emerged a set of ten principles that have come to be known as the Nuremberg Code (1948). These principles established the boundaries of human experimentation, clearly spelling out the degree to which moral and ethical considerations hold sway over the pursuit of scientific knowledge. The first of these principles is worth reproducing in full:

> The voluntary consent of the human subject is absolutely essential. . . . This means that the person involved should have legal capacity to give consent; should be so situated as to be able to exercise free power of choice, without the intervention of any element of force, fraud, deceit, duress, overreaching, or other ulterior form of constraint or coercion; and should have sufficient knowledge and comprehension of the elements of the subject matter as to enable him to make an understanding and enlightened decision. This latter element requires that, before the acceptance of an affirmative decision by the experimental subject, there should be made known to him the nature, duration and purpose of the experiment; the method and means by which it is to be conducted; all inconveniences and hazards reasonably to be expected; and the effects upon his health or person which may possibly come from his participation in the experiment.
>
> The duty and responsibility for ascertaining the quality of the consent rests upon each individual who initiates, directs,

> or engages in the experiment. It is a personal duty and responsibility which may not be delegated to another with impunity.

The other principles refer to such issues as prior animal experimentation, the "good of society," the avoidance of all unnecessary physical or mental suffering, the qualifications of the scientist, and the freedom of the subject to terminate the experiment at will.

Following this code, the World Medical Association adopted a set of rules on human experimentation in 1955; these were rewritten in 1961. In 1964, the same organization codified its principles on human experimentation in the Declaration of Helsinki. Thus, beginning in 1946, with the standards adopted by the American Medical Association, and continuing with the Nuremberg Code and the principles accepted by the World Medical Association in the 1950s and early 1960s, medical research was increasingly alerted to the ethical issues involved in human experimentation, and in particular, to the limits within which such research could be carried out.

An examination of the medical literature of the last one hundred and fifty years indicates that the moral and ethical obligation of physicians to serve the interests of their patients has been enunciated repeatedly. Thomas Percival in the early 19th century noted that "every rash experiment . . . is in the eye of conscience, a crime both against God and man." Somewhat later in the nineteenth century, a code of ethics was developed by the American Institute of Homeopathy, an organization of physicians involved in early efforts to develop vaccinations. This group pointed out:

> It is the physician's duty to state the true nature and prospects of the case, from time to time, to some judicious friend or relative of the patient, and to keep this person fully informed of the changes and probable issue. . . . The patient has the right to know the truth.

In areas of experimentation, where treatment was not the issue, the need to provide accurate and adequate information to the experimental subjects was an early consideration. One example was the work at the turn of the century of Walter Reed, who, in carrying out his yellow fever experiments, took careful steps to obtain written voluntary consent from the soldiers who had participated in the experiments. As described by Dr. Howard A. Kelly in his book *Walter Reed and Yellow Fever*, "Dr. Reed talked over the matter with them [the volunteers], explaining fully the danger and suffering involved in the experiment should it be successful, and then, seeing they were determined, he stated that a definite money compensation would be made to them." In 1948, a special advisory committee to the governor of Illinois emphasized ethical considerations with respect to the use of prisoners as experimental subjects. By the middle of the 20th century, the legal and medical literature was filled with examples that illustrate both the concern surrounding procedures that deviate from the norm as well as the importance attached to the requirements for disclosure and consent.

In 1966, in what was probably one of the century's most important papers on medical ethics in research, Henry K. Beecher, who was Dorr Professor of Research in Anesthesia at Harvard Medical School, called the profession to task for allowing the development since World War II of experimental research in which patients were either unwittingly subjected to research protocols or else never had the risks of the procedures adequately explained. He limited his discussion to those "areas of experimentation on a patient not for his benefit but for that, at least in theory, of patients in general." He expressed his concern about the inadequacy of existing forms of informed consent, as well as the ethics of some of the research protocols. He cited fifty studies that were problematic, and an examination of the work associated with these indicated that a further 186 might also be of concern. He graphically described twenty-two of the fifty studies and concluded that professional journals should refuse to publish the results of such studies. Beecher noted that in 1953 the Medical Research Council of Great Britain circulated a memorandum which suggested that publications had the obligation to make clear that the proprieties of disclosure and consent had been scrupulously observed. This implied that editors had some responsibility in the control of unethical human experimentation. Beecher strongly indicated, however, that the most important safeguard was the presence of a scientist of integrity.

This paper, published in *The New England Journal of Medicine*, caused quite a stir. In a book published the following year titled *Human Guinea Pigs: Experimentation on Man*, Pappworth described a similar process that he had been observing for many years in England. In addition, he described the great resistance on the part of scientific journal editors and medical professionals not only to listen to reports of ethical abuse but also to publicize concerns about the problem. Pappworth describes how clinical medicine over the 1950s and early 1960s became dominated by teaching and research hospitals. The issue then began to revolve around whether care was designed for individual patients and their illnesses or whether the treatment of an individual patient was a reflection of the current lines of research of that particular institution.

Pappworth quotes a distinguished British surgeon, Sir William Heneage Ogilvie, in 1952:

> The science of experimental medicine is something new and sinister; for it is capable of destroying in our minds the old faith that we, the doctors, are the servants of the patients whom we have undertaken to care for, and, in the minds of the patients, the complete trust that they can place their lives or the lives of their loved ones in our care.

In the same year, Pope Pius XII, in a talk at the First International Congress of Neuropathology, commented:

> Where does the doctor find a moral limit in research into and use of new methods and procedures in the "interests of the patient"? The limit is the same as that for the patient. It is that which is fixed by the judgment of sound reason. . . .

We can see, then, that despite the codes of ethics that had been established by this time, some physicians were ignoring widely accepted ethical principles and devoting themselves to research protocols that were unethical and utilized unwitting hospitalized patients as research subjects.

Distinctions have been made between what is termed therapeutic and nontherapeutic experimentation. Therapeutic experimentation is that which may have direct benefit to the patient, although the intervention is part of a research protocol designed to benefit a class of patients; nontherapeutic experimentation designates those procedures that differ from standard medical treatments and are designed principally to generate new knowledge. In the first category, subjects usually suffer from a specific illness that requires amelioration, whereas in the second, subjects more often tend to be normal. As well, in therapeutic experimentation, doctors appear to be hesitant to influence the decisions of their patients by alluding to experimental procedures; in nontherapeutic experimentation, a more open attitude to consent seems to exist. Yet this distinction is unreasonable, as Alexander Capron points out:

> The "normal volunteer" solicited for an experiment is in a good position to consider the physical, psychological, and monetary risks and benefits to him when he consents to participate. How much harder that is for the patient to whom an experimental technique is offered during a course of treatment! The man proposing the experiment is one to whom the patient may be deeply indebted for past care (emotionally as well as financially) and on whom he is probably dependent for his future well-being. . . .

It would appear that in Ewen Cameron's work at the Allan Memorial Institute, the line between therapy and research became blurred. Routine clinical intervention became extended increasingly so that treatment became experimental procedure, and the line between the two disappeared altogether. What confounds the situation even further is that Cameron's ambitions were so paramount that they eroded the physician-patient relationship. The trust that patients put in their doctor was misused; the needs of individual patients were subsumed in the overall goal. If one reads Cameron's work, especially the paper on sensory deprivation that was prepared for the 1964 San Antonio conference on that subject, it is clear that experimental procedures were being designed to further a theory of human behavior and to develop techniques of influencing behavior. Work was not concentrated on what was best for any one patient but on fashioning a methodology for behavioral change that would be applicable to a general class of patients. This is human experimentation, pure and simple. In notes made for this paper on March 18, 1960, Cameron reveals the progression of his thinking:

> Regarding sensory deprivation, make reference to the following:
> 1. My own work on nocturnal delirium
> 2. The early deprivation experiments (Allan)
> 3. The experiments on chemical deprivation
> 4. The special instance of Sernyl (PCP)—a sensory input block
> 5. The present sensory deprivation experiments
> 6. Projected experiments using drugs
> 7. Old experiments using ECT to break up the space-time image
> 8. Old experiments using LSD-25 for the same purpose
> 9. Also in paper, make reference to input-overload in terms of 1) sound 2) light 3) pain 4) verbal stimulation.

Thus, Cameron himself saw his work as experimentation. Further confirming that his procedures were not routine treatment are the following facts: he applied to, and received funding from, outside agencies to prove his theories, and he built a special laboratory in a separate part of the hospital to further his methodology.

An editorial in *The New England Journal of Medicine* following up on Beecher's paper on ethical experimentation decried the way that some unethical experimenters since Nuremberg had ignored the precepts of the Code. Cameron's research and consent procedures were not the standard of the time; however, he was in the company of a minority of researchers who were carrying out unethical experimentation on human subjects without informed consent. It is my opinion that his ambition and drive so clouded his sensitivities that he abused the trust of his patients; they became to him not humans in pain, but laboratory animals to be exploited in a search for the cure to mental illness. In that sense, there is a parallel with the Nazi physicians; their drive for the progress of science, as they so defined it, led them to dehumanize those on whom they worked. Their work was not only sanctioned but promoted by the state. It now appears that Cameron's work was similarly encouraged by the governments of two countries.

Cameron's experiments represent just one example of how government can contribute to unethical research. The involvement of the government of the United States in immoral work was brought to the attention of American citizens with the shocking revelation in 1972 that, for some forty years, the Public Health Service of the United States had been conducting a study on the long-term effects of untreated syphilis. The so-called Tuskegee Study was established in 1932 in a rural area of Alabama. Its purpose is shrouded in lack of clear documentation; however, we do know that it was designed to examine what the course of untreated syphilis would be in 399 poor black men, with another 201 black men serving as controls. Only men with late-stage syphilis were selected. For the next four decades, blood testing was done on these men, and autopsies were performed on the remains of the large number who died of tertiary syphilis. As of 1969, it was reported that somewhere between 28 and 100 men had died from the illness.

How was it that almost four hundred men would agree to allow themselves to suffer the ravages of a disease that ultimately can affect most of the organs of the body—a disease that can cause disfigurement, cardiovascular disease, and even dementia? James Jones, in his book *Bad Blood: The Tuskegee Syphilis Experiment*, describes graphically a heinous example of misguided medical adventurism. The men were primarily illiterate; this was the rural South in the midst of the Depression. They were offered many free services—physical examinations, transportation to the clinics, hot meals when examined, treatment for their medical ills (other than the syphilis), and, most important, burial stipends. Although there is no documentation concerning such issues as consent, it appears that these men were told very little. Jones reports that one of the men was told merely that he had "bad blood," and that he was being studied for this problem through the years.

When the study was made public, the Public Health Service officials tried to evade responsibility in many ways. For example, they indicated that at the time that the study was begun, treatment for syphilis was archaic and involved the use of dangerous compounds. They contended that the use of these substances could have been very dangerous. They did not explain why wealthier and white men and women were offered this treatment all over the world. In fact, it subsequently was revealed that some of the black men had in fact received modified forms of this treatment, thereby contaminating the results that would have been obtained from the experiment. Even more serious was the fact that in the 1940s, penicillin had become available—for the first time, syphilis could now be cured. Penicillin was not offered to all the black men, but it was offered to some, often for other complaints. Since this, too, would have affected the results, any conclusions from such a study were therefore highly suspect.

With cavalier disregard, the Public Health Service dismissed concerns about the study. Aspects of the work were published in many scientific journals and no one in the profession ever criticized the study—in fact, it had been approved by the local medical society. Jones describes how an official of the Public Health Service "pointed to a generation gap as a reason to refrain from criticizing it. 'We are trying to apply 1972 medical treatment standards to those of 1932.' " Jones continues:

> Another officer reminded the public that the study began when attitudes toward treatment and experimentation were much different. "At this point in time," the officer stated, "with our current knowledge of treatment and the disease and the revolutionary change in approach to human experimentation, I don't believe the program would be undertaken."

These are the same arguments that are espoused in the

Cooper Report and are nothing more than a whitewash, an attempt to deny culpability.

As the years went by, an occasional physician either within or outside the Public Health Service would begin to question the study, but many physicians responded to the press reports of the time by defending the experimentation. It was, as Jones indicates, defended on "a time-honored principle of the medical profession; namely, that 'good medicine' in any community is defined by the physicians who practice there." However, questions of racial prejudice began to surface for the first time. Once again, a disadvantaged group, in this instance, poor and black, had been exploited by medical researchers. Nazi prisoners, mental patients, poor black men—those that society labels as undesirable—are fringe members of a society and as such become vulnerable to abuse.

Shortly after the study was publicized, an ad hoc advisory panel was established by Merlin Du Val, an assistant secretary of Health, Education and Welfare. The final report of the panel appeared in April 1973; its findings are critically important to our consideration of the work at the Allan Memorial Institute.

> In retrospect, the Public Health Service Study of Untreated Syphilis in the Male Negro in Macon County, Alabama was ethically unjustified in 1932. . . . One fundamental ethical rule is that a person should not be subjected to avoidable risk of death or physical harm unless he freely and intelligently consents. There is no evidence that such consent was obtained from participants in the study.

Jay Katz, professor of psychiatry and law at Yale University, was a member of that panel. Feeling that the conclusions were not stated strongly enough, he wrote a concurring opinion that even more clearly attributes blame. He says:

> In theory, if not in practice, it has long been "a principle of medical and surgical mortality [never to perform] on man an experiment which might be harmful to him to any extent, even though the result might be highly advantageous to science" (Claude Bernard, 1865), at least without the knowl-

> edgeable consent of the subject. This was one basis on which the German physicians who had conducted medical experiments in concentration camps were tried by the Nuremberg Military Tribunal for crimes against humanity. . . . In conclusion, I note sadly that the medical profession, through its national association, its many individual societies and its journals, has on the whole not reacted to this study [the Tuskegee Syphilis experiment] except by ignoring it. . . . When will we take seriously our responsibilities, particularly to the disadvantaged in our midst who so consistently throughout history have been the first to be selected for human research?

In 1974, after a class action suit, the United States government settled with survivors and family members for $10 million. If legal action had not been taken, it is likely that redress would never have been achieved.

During the early years of this century, the courts began to raise the issue of consent, especially if the procedure could be construed in any way as a deviation from customary practice. Thus Justice Benjamin N. Cardozo in 1914 stated:

> Every human being of adult years and sound mind has a right to determine what shall be done with his own body; and a surgeon who performs an operation without his patient's consent commits an assault for which he is liable in damage.

And in another case in 1935 Cardozo said:

> We recognize the fact that, if the general practice of medicine and surgery is to progress, there must be a certain amount of experimentation carried on; but such experiments must be done with the knowledge and consent of the patient or those responsible for him, and must not vary too radically from the accepted method of procedure.

In *Informed Consent to Human Experimentation: The Subject's Dilemma*, George Annas and colleagues note that the first court decision on medical ethics was as far back as 1895, when the Colorado Supreme Court ruled that:

> If a physician sees fit to experiment with some other mode,

> he should do so at his peril. In other words, he must be able, in the case of deleterious results, to satisfy the jury that he had reason for the faith that was in him, and justify his experiment by some reasonable theory.

They cite two further cases. The Washington Supreme Court made the following ruling in 1902:

> [The physician] must not experiment in his treatment of the injury. On the contrary, if he desires to avoid liability for his mistakes, he must treat it in some method recognized and approved by his profession as the most likely to produce favorable results.

In a New York court case of 1941, the issue of consent is mentioned: "Initiative and originality should not be thus effectively stifled, especially when undertaken with the patient's full knowledge and consent, and as a last resort."

Jay Katz, in his informative book *The Silent World of Doctor and Patient*, has reviewed the history of informed consent as a legal doctrine. He emphasizes that, although by 1957 the AMA supported full disclosure and consent, medicine has always operated as a paternalistic and authoritarian profession. Physicians have reserved for themselves the right to decide how much a patient should be told. Often this was couched in terms of the physician's fear that the truth would disturb the patient too much, or at other times, truth was withheld because of biases on the part of the physician, such as racial or class prejudices. The courts in the United States have in a sense supported the physicians by formulating the conflict as "one about choosing liberty or caring custody." Katz notes that, historically,

> judges have made impassioned pleas for patient self-determination and then have undercut them by giving physicians considerable latitude to practice according to their own lights, exhorting them only to treat each patient with the utmost care.

In the 1950s, judges began to move from expecting doctors to disclose the nature of a procedure to asking whether patients have the right to weigh the costs and benefits of the intervention, and to decide if they want it. Although the courts had been addressing the issue of informed consent throughout this century, the doctrine was most clearly expressed on October 22, 1957 in the case of *Salgo vs. Leland J. Stanford, Jr. University Board of Trustees* before the California Court of Appeals. The case involved a man who became paralyzed after a procedure at Stanford designed to visualize the abdominal aorta through the injection of a dye and an X-ray process. Justice Bray's opinion is informative:

> A physician violates his duty to his patient and subjects himself to liability if he withholds any facts which are necessary to form the basis of an intelligent consent by the patient to the proposed treatment. . . . In discussing the element of risk, a certain amount of discretion must be employed with the full disclosure of facts necessary to an informed consent.

Katz makes the following very important point: "the justices might have been influenced by a line of cases, dating back at least to 1767, in which courts had warned physicians that, wherever they used new and as yet untried interventions, they did so 'at their peril.' " The Salgo case was thus a vivid clarification of the direction in which both the courts and organized medicine were moving during the 1940s and 1950s.

In 1960, in *Natanson vs. Kline*, Justice Schroeder of the Kansas Supreme Court promulgated the doctrine of self-determination—that decisions about the body can only be made by the individual whose body it is. In 1972, in *Canterbury vs. Spence*, Justice Robinson of the Washington, D.C. Circuit Court took away the tried and true defense of the profession, the defense of "customary practice": the procedure is deemed acceptable if it has been customarily practiced in the profession. "We sense the danger that what in fact is no custom at all," said Robinson, "may be taken as an affirmative custom to maintain silence. . . ."

The twists and convolutions that the doctrine of informed consent has taken in the courtroom reflect both the importance that judges have attached to the issue as well as their difficulty in assessing the proper role of the medical profession vis-à-vis their patients. To decide that patients have the right to full disclosure also means that judges must in fact fly in the face of historical precedent that places patients in a subordinate and compliant role with respect to their physicians.

I raise the issue of the development of legal precedents on the subject of informed consent because Ewen Cameron's patients did sign consent forms for treatment. These were the same forms that they would have signed if they had entered the Royal Victoria Hospital for gall bladder surgery or treatment of cystic acne. Although clear consent forms specifically for experimentation were in use during the late 1950s, this was not the case for Cameron's work at McGill. Cooper and Cameron's supporters within the medical profession would have us believe once again that this was standard for the times. But they are wrong. Both philosophically and historically, the medical profession has expected physicians to act with integrity and not to harm their patients. In addition, legal decisions both before and after the Nuremberg Code were moving physicians toward accepting informed consent as part of medical practice, and especially so with respect to human experimentation. Cameron's disregard for the rights of his patients, a disadvantaged group, was a reflection of a misuse of power that has appeared in certain elements of the profession since time immemorial.

During the 1950s there were no formal review processes in place at research settings to prevent a researcher from proceeding with even the most poorly designed or unethical experiment. However, at the government level, the Nuremberg Code was incorporated into policy decisions concerning experimentation even in the early 1950s. At the National Institutes of Health in Washington, D.C., the ethical requirement for consent was recognized by Dr. James M. McIntosh, a special consultant to the Public Health Service. A September 1952 memorandum from McIntosh to the director of the National Institute of Arthritis and Metabolic Diseases stated: "It is clear that the law would have to require . . . that the patient has been clearly informed of the nature and purpose of the experiment and of the results that it might involve. . . ."

Even the U.S. Army adopted the Nuremberg Code in 1953 as a basis for informed consent in human experimentation. The following year Irving Ladimer, an official with the National Institutes of Health, stated in a paper:

> Projects involving deviation from accepted medical practice or those in which unusual hazards lie are presented in writing and orally, to the Clinical Research Committee. . . . The Director of the National Institutes of Health must finally approve before patients or volunteer normal controls are permitted to participate after having demonstrated their full knowledge and consent.

In 1973, partially in response to the Tuskegee revelations, the National Institutes of Health appointed a special study group to review many of the issues that we have been addressing. This study group produced a document entitled "Protection of Human Subjects: Policies and Procedures." This was the first attempt to delineate policies that would ensure that no one, especially disadvantaged groups, could be exploited in the name of scientific research. In 1974 the United States Congress passed a National Research Act that established a National Commission for the Protection of Human Subjects in Biomedical and Behavioral Research. Since then, federal guidelines on conduct of research have been offered and amended several times over the years. In Canada, following much discussion, guidelines were established in 1978 for ethical conduct of research. Those applying for grants from the Medical Research Council were obligated to follow the guidelines. Subsequently, according to the Cooper Report, these guidelines became the standard in Canada for the conduct of any research. In the United States, an institution such as a university that receives federal funding must file an assurance that research will adhere to federal standards. As well, institutions must establish Human Subjects Committees composed of individuals representing different disciplines. These committees meet regularly to review all new research proposals and to review preexisting or continuing projects. Ethical considerations are paramount, as is the establishment of conditions for informed consent; thus, consent forms must be shown to the committee as part of the review. The approval of this committee is essential prior to receipt of external funding.

Given this kind of rigorous review, it is highly doubtful that a proposal such as Cameron's would ever have passed an ethics committee as they are presently constituted. His work would have been criticized on the basis of its lack of theoretical basis and its poor research design, selection of subjects, lack of informed consent, inadequate safeguards, inadequate prior research on animals—the inadequacies are legion.

One other area of great concern is the responsibility of funding agencies—for the ethics of the proposed research and also for the conduct of the investigator. Cooper is quick to point out that the Canadian government agencies that funded Cameron did their best "within the context of the time" to ascertain that the work was reasonable. The Central Intelligence Agency, in a similar fashion, indicates that it was merely funding an ongoing program of research conducted by an established investigator. Both governments suggest that the funding agencies had little moral or ethical responsibility for the work that they were supporting. I find this argument difficult to understand. If I were to hire a known gunman to kill someone, would I not be culpable? I know his reputation; I pay for his services; he is going to carry out something that I want done, even though it is evil. The CIA went looking for Ewen Cameron because they had been following his work; they funded him from 1957 through 1960 because they knew that his experimental direction was built upon brainwashing procedures and his research extended the work of MKULTRA. The experiment was unethical from its inception, but questions of ethics never appear to have been raised. By invoking present-day standards, the funding agencies excuse their behavior on the grounds that these research review procedures were not yet in place. But Cooper himself indicates that there were review procedures commonly used at the time; if the reviewers fell down on the job, the Agency cannot be excused on the basis of newer ethical standards set down ten or twenty years later. By giving money to Ewen Cameron, both the CIA and the Canadian government took upon themselves responsibility for the lives of patients who became unwitting experimental subjects.

Human experimentation will always be an area of controversy. Clearly, the contributions to science, and indeed to our understanding of disease and its cures, have been immeasurably aided by our ability to carry out research on human subjects. It is also apparent that we must constantly raise questions about the philosophical, theological, and sociocultural aspects of our medical interventions. The ethics and morality of our research methodology, and indeed of the new directions that medicine follows with the aid of advanced technology, must be paramount in our concerns. We must learn from the past; we must never forget.

16

A Story With No End

Sometimes I have to stop and ask myself if all of this really happened. The memories, although vivid, become submerged in the stream of daily events: attending committee meetings, seeing patients, taking my children to soccer practice, doing the laundry, grocery shopping. Yet the multitude of tasks that encompass the boundaries of my life occupy only the foreground of the painting. Underneath, in murky tones of blue and gray, the background is always present, casting a pall but not quite seen. Reality intrudes with a vengeance when I receive a notice of deposition from the CIA attorneys—I am to appear with all of my notes, with all the chapters of the manuscript for this book, with copies of the many papers that I have photocopied. Yes, the events that engulfed my father did take place, and resolution of the tragedy seems an impossible fantasy.

When I think about the last few years, what stands out most clearly are the many people with whom I have spoken about the case. Lawyers, diplomats, physicians, former patients of Cameron, colleagues of Cameron. Many of them had strong opinions; all of them in some way had been touched by the man, his work, or the aftermath. There are rooms of elegance and spare rooms of genteel poverty; modern library reading rooms contrast with a dusty basement containing old file cabinets. Intense, patient hours slide into solitary hours in front of a word processor. Oftentimes this case has been the focus of my thoughts; perhaps I have occasionally been too preoccupied with all that I have learned. Yet as I have listened to the people I interviewed, as I have read about sensory deprivation and brainwashing, I have realized that the story is important, not only to me but to those of us who care about civil liberties and about those vulnerable individuals whom society finds it expedient to abuse.

A whole new dimension has opened in my life as I have learned about the news media. Television and radio reporters vary widely, both in their understanding of the human beings that provide the meat for their stories and in their ability to elicit compassionately from the interviewee the substance of his or her pain. As I have said, I was struck during the taping of one television program by the way in which the well-known interviewer changed from a warm and thoughtful man to an opinionated television "personality" when the camera was on. Radio producers would call from around the United States and Canada. After talking with them for twenty minutes and being impressed with their knowledge and concern, I would agree to take part in their program. At the appointed time, a totally strange individual would be put on the line to do the interview, someone with whom I had never spoken, and whom I could not see. "The interview will take three or four minutes, Dr. Weinstein." How does one convey the many issues? How can one communicate the anguish? How does one portray a character of evil intent? But I tried.

Newspaper reporters have been, on the whole, more systematic and thoughtful. Sometimes what has appeared in print, however, was not entirely as I had meant it to be. And then the Hollywood filmmakers began to telephone; they were enthusiastic and anxious to produce a film: "Has anyone signed up you or your father yet?" These people had called because of a small story, an item that caught their eye in a newspaper. I asked them to call again when they had reviewed all the facts, I suggested what to read. But I never heard from them. "Why do you waste your time talking to these people?" I am asked. "Because I want the world to know," I reply.

I am sitting in my office after one of these telephone calls. My patient is a young woman; she is very pretty, tall with long hair that catches the sunlight streaming in the window. She is a law student at one of the finest schools in the country, a Phi Beta Kappa graduate of an Ivy League college and the daughter of a wealthy Long Island family. She has been binge-eating and vomiting up her food three to four times a day for four years. In the mirror she sees only fat; no one, she thinks, can appreciate how ugly she really is. Her life is spent in pleasing others because, if she disagrees or asserts herself, they will surely reject her. And yet she cannot assert herself because she does not know what she feels. Her life is spent in reaction—to people, to situations, to expectations of disapproval. Who is she? I wonder.

As I listen to her describe her despair and loneliness, I think about the telephone call from Hollywood. For a while I tune into my patient and, at the same time, I listen to the currents of my life. We are not alone in the room: her parents, friends, and lovers circulate through a crowd of my old friends and my parents; reporters take notes as Ewen Cameron walks into the room, surrounded by his residents. I feel sad; anger awakens. My patient tells me that she wants to die; life has no meaning. In my reverie, a woman enters the room—her ears are covered with special earphones, goggles hide her eyes. She is led to a doorway where a bed and a darkened room await. For a while we are surrounded by pain, and then a trio of musicians enters; it is my grandfather and two of his cronies dressed as they did in the *shtetl* of Eastern Europe. A sweet melody fills the air, "Romania, Romania. . . ." The hour draws to a close. I have heard every word that my patient has told me; I have responded appropriately. She did not know that our conversation took place in the midst of a crowd; she did not hear me; she does not know me. That is the way of psychotherapy. I am alone.

In February 1986, Florence Langleben, one of the nine Canadians suing the CIA, died of cancer in Florida. Although she was only sixty-nine years of age, her death came as a cruel reminder of the length of time that it has taken for these Canadians to have their day in court. The *Montreal Gazette* said in an editorial:

> The death of this Montreal woman is still a shocking reminder of the Canadian government's craven indifference to the plight of people who shared her experience. . . . The case has been bogged down in pre-trial procedures in the U.S. for five years while U.S. and Canadian authorities exchange polite letters and try to cover their backsides behind national security arguments. . . .

The death of Mrs. Langleben also made me acutely aware both of my father's age (he was then eighty years old) and that of our lawyer, Joe Rauh, who was in his seventy-sixth year. A victim had died with the fight just begun. Were these former patients to be dogged by powerlessness until they passed on? The CIA has both the money and time to drag the case out for years; we can afford neither of those luxuries. In fact, the CIA has made it clear that if it were to lose this suit in the District Court of Washington, D.C., it has every intention of appealing right up to the Supreme Court if necessary. Yet we all continue to act as though the day in court is imminent, and that resolution is possible. Why do we do this? For me, the opportunity to reveal the machinations of the CIA (and of the Government of Canada) vindicates my father; for him, he at last feels a sense of efficacy; for the attorneys, not only do they fight for the lives of their clients, but they are committed to the preservation of civil liberties in the United States. What, however, can I say to the former patient of Cameron who is so destitute that life is a hand-to-mouth existence?

December 1986. A letter arrives from Rauh's law offices. As usual, I feel a flood of anxiety when I open the envelope; this time, my worst fears are confirmed. My eyes are riveted on one word, "Farewell." Goodbye, so long, it is over. I had suspected for several months that Joe Rauh was feeling his age. Arthritis in his hips had forced him to use a cane, tennis games became memories, and at times a fleeting shadow of pain would cross his craggy features as he shifted in his chair or walked. No, I was not surprised, but an immeasurable amount of sadness descended upon me. I was not concerned about the future conduct of the case from the legal perspective; I had something greater to lose. Joe Rauh had given me something priceless. In his tenacity, his gutsy determination to see the case through to conclusion, in his ability to focus on the vulnerabilities of poor logic, Joe had assumed the role of father for me. He had stepped into the void of thirty years and helped me once again to stand up straight. True, the relationship had not been unambivalent; relationships with fathers seldom are. At times I had disagreed with him; at times I had been in awe of his intellect. But always I had respected him. For me, the loss was significant. The gift that was given to me on a personal basis was far greater than any that could have come to me through the legal process. I will never forget him.

March 1987. Judge Penn has just heard arguments concerning the motion of the CIA to have the case dismissed. It will take a while to hear the outcome of this latest round. My father has arrived for his yearly trip to California.

He is sitting in the sun, protected from the wind off the ocean by his old blue trenchcoat. My son's San Francisco Forty-Niner hat is pulled down over my father's brow; from his mouth, the omnipresent cigar dangles. The slightly bitter penetrating smell destroys the fresh honey scent of a California meadow in spring glory. He does not know that I am watching.

He is an old man; the realization dawns on me as if I simply hadn't noticed. The gray hair is even thinner than it was eight months ago; he sleeps more, catnaps have lengthened into a dream-filled respite from thoughts of the past. He looks like his sisters before they died, I think. The thought of death chills me as I wonder how much time is left; what more must he and I go through before he finally finds peace? My sons are on the floor playing a game, filled with laughter, fighting, and the loving rivalry of twinship. My father sits under the clear sky; I stand in the doorway;

my sons, blissfully unaware of mortality. Three generations bound together—fathers and sons. What will I bequeath to my children? Through how many generations does pain extend? What longings will they have? A chain of men loving and hating, accepting and fighting, confronting the world that was and is.

I leave and walk along the cliff. Past, present, and future whirl in my mind as I let the realization sink in—he is old. There is not much time left. The waves pound the rocks, the images pound my brain, and I let myself go. Inside the anger builds—like the cigar, an alien scent in this place of such beauty. The purple of wild iris, the gold of poppies, the green of the rain-drenched meadows. I walk aware and detached, living my life as I always have, as participant and observer. What is left but to fight? There is no other choice for me.

Ahead lies the possibility of a trial, and I think about the issues on which it will focus. These are the concerns that the CIA has raised as it steadfastly maintains its innocence. First, the notion is presented that Ewen Cameron was a great man, an eminent psychiatrist; a man they could rely upon. If so, the logic goes, how can he have carried out work that was unethical? How could such a great man have done such a thing? It is quite apparent that Cameron was sufficiently prominent that the nine patients, and indeed many others, went to him for treatment. What this reasoning ignores, however, is the simple fact that Cameron's fame was not built on his abilities as a researcher—where he was mediocre—but on his considerable strengths as a politician. Second, as we have seen from the Nuremberg trials, from the revelations of Tuskegee, and from the concerns expressed by Beecher, supposedly eminent men were very capable of being unethical. They were eager, in fact, to take advantage of those who could not question—prisoners, mental patients, poverty-stricken and illiterate black men. Fame and reputation do not necessarily confer honor or integrity.

Testimony is sought from colleagues of Cameron that seems to excuse his behavior on the basis of his zeal to cure. Thus, what begins as noble compassion becomes a laudable mission. It then becomes entangled with ambition until patient needs become secondary to the fulfillment of a messianic dream. How can such rationalizations make Cameron's behavior acceptable? Since when do we downplay the significance of such dangerous blind spots? There is great consistency in descriptions of Cameron's personality—aloof, power driven, politically manipulative, and committed to his career. Where there is dispute is in the extent of his commitment to his patients. Was he in fact desirous of helping them as individuals, or was he seeking a Nobel Prize? Was it their individual concerns that moved him, or was he pushed by a missionary zeal that said, "I will make you better for your own good—whether you like it or not, your disease will yield to me." Most of the data unfortunately suggests that the latter explanation is the more likely.

The second proposal offered in Cameron's defense is that his work was acceptable within the standard of the time. It is quite true that electroconvulsive therapy, insulin comas, and the use of barbiturates and amphetamines were widely employed in treatment. However, regressive shock treatment was not a generally accepted treatment program; LSD had been experimented with, but not in combination with all of the other drugs that were part of Cameron's package; sleep treatment was used in modified form in the USSR where it had evolved, and in a few places in Europe, but once again, not for such prolonged periods of time nor in concert with these other approaches. The Russian pioneer of the sleep-therapy approach, B. V. Andreev, reported that in his group of patients sleep usually lasted for ten to thirteen hours, and occasionally for fourteen to fifteen hours, with an average duration of one to three weeks.

It is a fact that nowhere else in the world but at the Allan was sensory deprivation used to treat patients. The bizarre cocktails of PCP, LSD, curare, barbiturates, amphetamines, nitrous oxide, and insulin coma—given in sequence to the same patient—were not standard treatment in any civilized country. The unique process of psychic driving that Cameron offered psychiatry was not an intervention that was used in any other setting. The hours of recorded messages would not have been inflicted on these patients if they had been fortunate enough to receive treatment at any other institution in Canada or the United States. They were, however, techniques of interest to the CIA, and the similarity between Cameron's work and the brainwashing techniques of the Chinese Communists is striking. The parallels are too close to be coincidence. These methods were hardly the standard of the time for psychiatry; perhaps they were for interrogators.

The issue of informed consent is another that emerges in the CIA's defense of its innocence. Cameron's blanket consent form, it is suggested, was also "standard for the time." It is quite apparent that specific consent forms for experimental subjects were in active use during the 1950s when explicit experimental procedures were being tried. Francis D. Moore, in "Biologic and Medical Studies in Human Volunteer Subjects: Ethics and Safeguards," emphasizes the need for "a signed and witnessed permission slip that is completely realistic in all its details." He goes on to describe the need for utmost specificity. This paper was published in 1960 and presumably written and discussed before that time. We have also discussed earlier how both the medical profession as well as the courts had produced documents that indicated the need for informed consent by the time that Ewen Cameron began his program of research in the mid-1950s. So much for this leg of the CIA's defense.

Another point that has been raised—this time in the Cooper Report—is the issue that Cameron published his work and no one raised a fuss. Therefore, it must have been acceptable. Yet no one over the ten years that Cameron carried out his work adopted or replicated it at other institutions. Even two of the three expert witnesses upon whom Cooper relied had grave reservations at the time. How is it that Cameron's colleagues kept silent? It may have been his power and that old bugaboo, "eminence." But how do we explain other cases—Alabama, Nazi Germany, the fifty cases cited by Beecher—where medical doctors remained mute in the face of horrible acts committed by their colleagues. Does all this represent a weakness in the profession? Does science and the quest for truth blind physician-researchers to issues of morality? I do not know the answer to these questions, but I do know that the statement "but no one protested" is an unreasonable way to dismiss guilt. There are too many precedents where the same argument was used to hide the truth.

More specifically, the CIA has claimed that Cameron began this work long before they became involved with him, and that the Government of Canada provided funding long before them. They were just helping a scientist who was doing work in which they were interested. But Gittinger has testified that the CIA *invited* Cameron to submit a grant application. The agency also gave Cameron a considerable amount of money to enable him to develop more sophisticated methods, both of breaking people down and of reprogramming them. We have seen how his work not only mirrored that of other recipients of MKULTRA funding but indeed carried it significantly further. CIA funding was not incidental to the program.

We are therefore left with a situation in which a well-known psychiatrist developed and declared himself responsible for a program of research in which a vulnerable group of people, his patients, were hurt. Some have wondered why the patients or their families did not question; other psychiatrists make allusions to the "strong positive transference" that some of the women patients must have had for this man. I believe that there is a very simple explanation for both of the above. Since Cameron's power could intimidate his colleagues, how could it do less to his patients and their families? He abused the physician-patient relationship; his stance of omnipotence and omniscience placed his patients in a position of such helplessness that, to this day, many are tormented by the shame of the degradation that was their lot. To make their acquiescence a reflection of their supposed psychopathology demonstrates again that, once stigmatized, a vulnerable group of people faces an uphill battle to regain respect and equality.

Some have suggested that one reason for the relative lack of public outcry around this case has been the fact that the events occurred roughly thirty years ago. This is all in the past, they say, nothing like MKULTRA can happen again; Red-baiting was a symbol of a political climate long gone.

Yet it is unfortunately true that, since the era of the *mea culpa* openness of the intelligence establishment that took place during the tenure of Admiral Turner as the CIA director and Jimmy Carter as president, there has been an increasing reversion to secrecy—a perfect example being the Iran-Contra affair. Furthermore, the atmosphere of the 1950s *has* returned. Under the Reagan administration, Red-baiting resurfaced and military preparedness became an obsession. In these circumstances, how can we be so sure that MKULTRA-type programs are things of the past?

Given the climate of the times, it is not surprising that, in the case of the Canadian plaintiffs, the CIA is holding to its assertion that it bears only incidental responsibility. Supported by the 1985 Supreme Court decision that the CIA did not have to reveal the names of its researchers, and by further decisions that protect CIA information under the guise of national security, the agency is buttressed in its intent to stand firm. The Reagan administration, in its support of the intelligence services, reverted to a position that we have not seen in the United States for many years. The response to this case by the United States government would likely have been significantly different during the 1970s.

Gray gothic buildings and a leaden sky; a biting wind that seems to sweep down from Hudson's Bay cutting into me; icy fingers massaging the wound that does not close. I stand at the top of the steps and look out over Ottawa. So many memories as I climb to the entrance—another stone building, other bleak days—and once again I feel very small as I prepare to confront those in authority. It is December 1987. I am in Canada's capital city, here to participate in a concerted effort to force the politicians to acknowledge responsibility. The case is now going into its eighth year. Two weeks before, when I had called Jim Turner in Washington for an update, he told me that messages were going back and forth between Ed Broadbent, leader of the NDP in Canada, and Minister of Justice Ray Hnatyshyn, about a proposal that was buried in the appendix of the Cooper Report. Cooper had suggested that the Canadian government, given the tragedy that had taken place, might offer an *ex gratia* payment of $100,000 to each of the plaintiffs. This payment, while not admitting any responsibility, would indicate the concern of the government that Canadian citizens had suffered in this manner.

Both Broadbent and Svend Robinson, another member of Parliament and the NDP justice critic, had been actively attempting to bring Cooper's proposal to fruition. They were not merely supporting this idea out of party loyalty. Both men acted out of a conviction that an injustice had occurred—one in which the Government of Canada had clearly participated.

On the day that I called Turner, he had received word that the offered payment was likely to be $20,000 per plaintiff. This figure, which was suspiciously similar to that offered earlier by the CIA to rid themselves of the nuisance of a court proceeding, was not only insulting but demeaned the very lives of those who had suffered. After some discussions with Orlikow, Broadbent, and Robinson, a decision had been reached to have a press conference, to ask questions on the floor of the House of Commons, and to have the plaintiffs write an open letter to the prime minister. I felt that I ought to be there when all of this took place, and so on December 10 I found myself in Ottawa on Parliament Hill. Turner had arranged for three of the plaintiffs to be present as well: Mr. Page, Mme. Jeanine Huard, and Mrs. Orlikow would all attend. Although I knew Mme. Huard well, I had not met the other two, both of whom had been very active in their attempts to move the case forward in Canada.

For me, this was my first foray into Canadian political life, and as I entered the Parliament Building my feelings were a mixture of anticipation and fear. I was excited at the possibility of confronting the enemy (for so I now thought of them) on their own territory, and at the same time, I was afraid that the outcome would be nothing more than a repetition of the disappointments that had stalked our lives for so long.

The stone lobby of Parliament was ablaze with Christmas lights and smelled of pine and spruce. I was assailed by sensations—smell, light, the sounds of the security men as they checked me for metal; internal sensations of excitement, of pain, of being on the brink—on the edge of what? I did not know.

I left the elevator and met Jim Turner outside David Orlikow's office. Out of his law office, and in the halls of Parliament, he seemed strangely out of place; he felt very American, and I felt myself become very Canadian. He, too, must have noticed a cultural disparity, because he remarked on how different Washington was from Ottawa. Disparate strands of my life seemed to be coming together, and the tension was so great that I almost could not move.

He showed me the open letter that had been delivered to the prime minister that morning; it was to be followed by a press conference and questions to the minister of justice by Svend Robinson. The letter ended as follows: "How many more of us must die, before Canada does what is right and fulfills its many promises to help us?" Sad words from powerless people—would they have any effect at all?

As I was sitting with Jim, Mr. and Mrs. Orlikow came in. David Orlikow is a short, unassuming man whose interests are broad and whose knowledge about a wide range of subjects is very impressive. His commitment to Canada and to the ideals of the NDP make him a champion of those whose basic rights are at risk. It seemed somehow ironic to me that a man whose professional life was devoted to caring about and protecting the average citizen was to have his personal life so bound up in the powerlessness of shielding a loved one from the anonymity of government muscle.

Mrs. Orlikow is a brave woman. Outgoing, at times abrasive, she radiates a warmth that alternates with a feisty determination to rectify the injustice that was done to her. I had seen her on television and so had formed an opinion of what she would be like. She had clearly been affected by the Cameron experiments. Her life could have been a shambles, but she made the most of what was left. In order to effect a sense of order and control, she took command—a veneer that hid a core of despair and dependency. I responded to her gutsy determination at once.

Mme. Huard was her usual gracious self—at one and the same time in control and fragile. I learned that she had recently moved to a small apartment as she could no longer afford to keep up her house. Mr. Page was very anxious; he was the most visibly wounded.

So here was our group—three of Cameron's victims: two family members whose lives had been irrevocably changed by the events of thirty years ago, and the attorney on whom so many hopes rested.

Lunch was in the Parliamentary Dining Room. It seemed somehow incongruous to be sitting there in that gracious setting—the Christians having tea in the boudoir of the lions. Mrs. Orlikow acted as the perfect hostess. Svend Robinson came over to say hello. I could not eat; knowing that I was to speak at a press conference took my appetite away. Suddenly, I caught my breath. The prime minister had entered; with practiced ease, he made his way from table to table (shades of my father) and finally settled in a corner. I saw Mrs. Orlikow change; suppressed anger emerged as she gave vent to her feelings, putting into words what we all felt. She soon regained her composure and we returned to comments about the salmon and the view of the Ottawa River. The split between living in the present and dealing with the past, between pleasantries and internal rage, was never more apparent than at that meal.

The press conference was held across the street at the National Press Club. As we entered, it was suddenly apparent to me that I was to be on the dais with Turner and Robinson. Svend Robinson would lead off. The others took seats in the first row. I do not know if it was the fact that the free-trade agreement was to be announced that day, or if reporters were tired of the story, but only five or six were present in the big room. Two television networks were also there. I felt disappointed. When Robinson spoke, his words were confident and clearly put the onus on the government to explain how they could justify not making any payment to the plaintiffs. Jim talked, and then it was my turn. I had prepared a great deal of material, but the emphasis appeared to be on the personal experience once again. I tried to talk about organic damage, of permanent impairment, but I am not certain that anyone heard. The three plaintiffs were asked about their experiences—and then it was over. The story was picked up by the Canadian press and some local newspapers. That was it.

I felt drained. I was concerned about the effect of this great stress on Mr. Page, Mme. Huard, and Mrs. Orlikow. We moved on to the House of Commons, where we were given reserved seats in the gallery. Down on the floor of the House, the players in the drama of Canadian political life were emoting for their constituents and each other. We were facing the prime minister, the justice minister, and others in the Cabinet. I wanted to stand and shout, "Wait! Some Canadians are hurting. Stop the pain." On the floor, the members of Parliament were attacking the health minister because shellfish from Prince Edward Island was tainted, and several people had become mortally ill. Free trade, poisoned shellfish, and images of the past—to what would the members of Parliament respond?

From *Hansard*, December 10, 1987:

> Mr. Svend Robinson (Burnaby): Mr. Speaker, my question is for the Minister of Justice. As the Minister knows, in the later 1950s a number of Canadians were victims of terrible brainwashing experiments by Dr. Ewen Cameron in Montreal, funded both by the Canadian government and the CIA. In view of the permanent scars that were suffered by these individuals, a number of whom are suing the CIA and, in fact, a number of whom are in the gallery today, when will the Minister do the right thing and offer each of these elderly victims an *ex gratia* payment of $100,000 to ease their burden, as was discussed in the Cooper Report last year?

In response, Mr. Hnatyshyn, the minister of justice and attorney general of Canada, reviewed the Cooper Report and its conclusion that "there is no legal liability on the part of the Government of Canada." He went on:

> I have been trying to do some negotiation and discussion with my colleagues, particularly with the Honourable Member for Winnipeg North [Orlikow] as an interlocutory between these people and the Government, to see if some assistance might

> be possible with respect to out of pocket expenses or legal costs that would be incurred.

Robinson replied that it was shameful that the government had found $650,000 to pay the legal fees of a Cabinet minister accused of wrongdoing and could not find any money to recompense the Cameron victims. He continued: "When will the Government finally do the right and decent thing and pay these people the compensation to which they are entitled before even more of the elderly victims have died? When will the Government finally act?"

The minister of justice noted that the government had compassion and that it would try to determine a reasonable amount of money that could be made available to the victims.

It was over. As we left the chamber, Robinson came out. There was some hubbub; Turner was pleased; Page was depressed; Mme. Huard was disappointed; Mrs. Orlikow was angry. I could feel the swirl of feelings around me—for the three victims, the hours provoked a roller-coaster sense of hope and despair. It was difficult for me; for them, it was almost unbearable. Robinson had spoken forthrightly and had represented these men and women well. What would the response of the government be?

Afterward, there was not much discussion. Clearly agitated, Mr. Page wanted to leave and return to his home near Montreal; Mrs. Orlikow and Mme. Huard wanted to go out for awhile; I remained with Turner and Orlikow. Another man had joined the group—Kalman Kaplansky was an old colleague of Orlikow, a trade unionist who had represented Canada in international organizations, a respected mediator and negotiator. We decided that a meeting with the deputy minister of justice was the next step. It was arranged for the following day; Kaplansky, Turner, and I would go.

The next morning, we walked to the minister's office. How far I had come since the days when I first began to question how my father's life had been ruined. The air was crisp; it had snowed the night before, and the white lawns glistened in the late autumn sun. Ottawa is a handsome city of stone buildings with green copper roofs. Its British heritage gives it a majesty that can be a little intimidating. And yet, it felt good to be on a "negotiating team," and I looked forward to the meeting.

We were ushered into the large office/conference room of the deputy minister, a gracious woman named Mary Dawson. There was something vaguely familiar about her. In the room were several others—some from the ministry of justice; others from the ministry of external affairs. One was the man who had collaborated on, and perhaps was the primary author of, the Cooper Report. He never spoke, but only took notes throughout the course of our long discussion. As I looked around the room, I noticed several diplomas on the wall. I was struck by the familiar McGill University style, and I suddenly realized that the deputy minister had been in my graduating class. She had gone through law school with many of my friends. When I commented on the diploma, she told me her maiden name. I thought that we had met, and she revealed that she was close to some of my old medical school classmates.

The friendly repartee ceased abruptly as the discussion began. Kalman Kaplansky reviewed his understanding of an *ex gratia* payment; basically, such a payment could be offered by the government as a token of concern without any admission of responsibility for what had transpired. Ms. Dawson and others noted that such a payment had been under active consideration for some time, but that she did not know where the minister now stood on the issue. We noted his comments on the floor of the House on the previous day and reiterated our understanding that he was amenable to this proposal. The conversation then focused, and eventually foundered, on what constituted a reasonable amount. It was the feeling of the government that the amount should be set at a level that could be used for payment of legal costs associated with bringing the CIA case to trial in Washington, D.C.; Turner pointed out that these were impoverished people to whom a significant sum of money would represent a lifeline. Another major area of disagreement was that we simply did not accept the final conclusion of Cooper's report, which held that the Government of Canada bore no responsibility for Cameron's work. When I emphasized this point, Ms. Dawson indicated that the report was not government policy; it was merely a legal opinion. I asked her why it was, then, that when American psychiatrists wrote to the minister of external affairs or to the justice minister, they received copies of the Cooper Report. If it were not policy, why was it used to substantiate the position of Canada? She did not reply.

As the talk continued, it became apparent that the government was quite concerned that if too great an amount were offered, it would open up government agencies to lawsuits, not only in this case but in other situations where government funding of research might have led to adverse consequences for experimental subjects. Such a precedent might be too dangerous. Clearly, the position of Canada was to make an offer in order to respond to the media and public interest, but also to contain this kind of demand by offering very little money so that others would not be tempted. We went back and forth; my erstwhile classmate had matured into the perfect government spokesperson. Her loyalties were clear; her emotions, well controlled. As the meeting drew to a close, it was apparent that an offer would be made within the month; the amount was still to be determined.

As I flew back to California, I suddenly felt very weary. Perhaps we had taken a small step, but the process had been taxing. How was it that all of those so involved in negotiating could have no empathy for the men and women who had spent weeks in isolation, listened to repetitive insults, having been drugged and shocked into vegetative states? I wished that I could take Mary Dawson back to my college years so that she could see the red leather couch on which lay a somnolent man, confused and irritable. I wished that she could have seen my mother age as she tried to reason with irrationality. How I wished that I could play a videotape of my memories in that room to force a recognition in complacent bureaucrats that people were destroyed—mothers, fathers, sons, and daughters.

It was the middle of January 1988. We had heard nothing directly, although one newspaper had quoted a source as indicating that the checks were ready to be signed by the appropriate government representative. On Tuesday, January 19, my office phone rang. It was Jim Turner calling from Washington, D.C.

"We won!" he yelled.

"What?" I wasn't sure to what he was referring.

He then told me that Judge Penn had made his decision on the CIA motion to throw the case out. He had decided that this case should go to trial in June. In addition, he felt that each of the plaintiffs should have their day in court, except Dr. Morrow, whose case had exceeded the statute of limitations.

I was elated. At last, after eight years, the debate would be carried out in open court, and we would have the opportunity to move beyond the news media and to air the considerable amount of evidence that had been gathered. When I put the receiver down, I began to cry. I felt the tension that had been built up in Ottawa and over the past year escape as a flood of sadness engulfed me. I wanted to run out of my office and yell, but who would be able to understand what this meant? When I called Rhona, my wife and I were for the first time filled with optimism that the case would be heard before my father died.

Ah, but the amusement park of life does not provide a ride that gives sustained pleasure. Lurking around the corner was the next horror; we were to be let down once again. Shortly after Judge Penn's decision was announced, my father received in the mail a check from the Government of Canada for $20,000. Ms. Dawson and her colleagues had followed through—they paid the nine plaintiffs a total of $180,000. this "magnanimous" gesture to Mme. Huard, who had been forced to sell her house; to Mr. Page, who lives on a minimal income; to my father, whose working life had ended abruptly at age 49; and to the others whose lives were destroyed was the ultimate cynical gesture of a government to its citizens.

On February 13 the *Montreal Gazette* commented in an editorial:

> The Canadian government has finally recognized some responsibility toward victims of brainwashing experiments at the Allan Memorial Institute nearly thirty years ago. The pity

> is that it has done so in a grudging, miserly, and inappropriate way . . . . [it is] almost an insult to their long struggle for justice.

More disappointments were to come. By the end of February, the CIA had adopted a stalling tactic that would require another decision on the part of Judge Penn. This raised the possibility that an Appeals Court would have to make a decision on whether the case should proceed. Once again, delay seemed inevitable.

Doubt. I awoke one morning and felt a sense of uncertainty. At first vague, as the day wore on it became a force that threatened to throw all my beliefs into question. All of us have moments when hard-fought convictions suddenly appear questionable, when all the energy that has been poured into a fight, a competition, a set of beliefs that identify who you are, seems somehow misplaced. I carried the doubt like a penitent; everywhere that I went, it ate away a part of myself. Like a parasite that lives while it destroys its host, the doubt blossomed as my energy fell. Going through the day became a chore, and I found it difficult to concentrate as my thoughts flitted from Washington to Ottawa to Montreal. Despite the depression, I forced myself to perform, but inside I felt as though my life spirit was draining away. This sadness persisted for several weeks until the words of a patient broke the slide.

A young woman with whom I had worked for several years had never been able to accept the loss of her father—first through divorce, then through premature death. His continued presence in her life had affected her relationships, her identity as a woman and as a competent professional; for her, this man had never left. And yet, he had never met her needs during his lifetime. In fact, many of her problems stemmed from her fruitless attempts to second-guess his expectations. Frustrated that she could never be perfect for him, she had lived her life in his shadow—afraid to risk, afraid to be at peace with herself. On this day she suddenly looked at me and commented: "You know, maybe I am better off that he is dead. Maybe I can go on with my life." Her eyes welled up with tears and I felt that a turning point had been reached.

I did not think very much about her words as the day passed, but apparently those tearful thoughts had triggered a response inside me that emerged at night in a dream.

I was walking down a street and turned into a walkway with a white gate. I opened it and saw my patient with a blue dog on a leash. As I moved forward, the dog attacked and ferociously began to eat away at my stomach. As I looked down, I realized that I was in great pain, and that part of me was disappearing into the jaws of the blue beast. I yelled at my patient: "Stop him! Can't you get him to stop?" She calmly said, "I can't, but you can. The dog is inside you."

I awoke sweating. The terror was real, and I could still feel the pain in my abdomen. What was the dream? What message was I receiving from the recesses of my brain? Relax and think; breathe slowly and try to understand. Blue—why a blue dog? It was a bright blue and I remembered that I was amazed at its color. Blue—I had been blue; it was depression that I was dreaming about. And the dog attacking me; it was inside me—the depression was inside eating away at my guts. My patient had made a significant breakthrough in letting go of her father and she was telling me to pay attention to how I was letting the governments of Canada and the United States, the CIA, and all those who made me doubt eat away at my beliefs. She was also telling me to let my father go; it was correct to fight for my beliefs, but I could not let memories of the tragedy destroy my life. I fell asleep and, in the morning, the depression had lifted. What remained was anger at the course of events. What had replaced the depression was a renewed determination to fight until some resolution was achieved—no matter how long it took.

In the early spring, Judge Penn again decided that the case must go to trial, and he set a court date of June 7. Shortly thereafter, I was informed that I would be called by the CIA to give my deposition on April 28. Little did I realize how intense an experience this would be. The deposition began at 10:00 A.M. and lasted until 8:00 P.M.; it continued the following day from 8:00 A.M. to 10:00 A.M.. I was informed that another day would be scheduled in the future since the questioning had not been completed. Although exhausted, I welcomed the advent of the forthcoming trial. But it was not to be. On May 20, the judge decided that the case would be postponed until October. An expert witness of the government had been seriously injured in an automobile accident, and the CIA also needed time to obtain other documentation. Judge Penn did, however, make the following comment in the postponement order: "The defendant is on notice, however, that the Court will look unfavorably on a future request for a continuance of the trial." In other words, Judge Penn put the CIA on notice that the trial had to begin in October. The waiting would soon be over.

The story of Cameron and his victims will not end. Whatever they may ultimately win—if they win at all—the nine Canadians have lost thirty years of living. Their children, spouses, and parents have been touched with a shadow that will not disappear. This is, most of all, a story of people; of love and friendship, respect and honor; of rage and despair. It is a tale of ambition and dishonor, of a profession whose weaknesses are all too apparent. Many lives have become interwoven in pursuit of the truth—my father's, mine, Ewen Cameron's, those of the attorneys, the other patients, politicians, reporters. The themes of ethical behavior, morality, secrecy, the contribution of the law to the regulation of medical practice—all of these make up the fabric of a piece of cloth dyed black.

Three years ago, I first began to collect articles that were relevant to Cameron's work. I found that, as months passed, more and more of my free time was devoted to thinking about the issues raised by the events at the Allan Memorial Institute. When I first began to write this book, I would find myself staring at the keyboard with wet cheeks. Memories would return with an intensity that could destroy my sense of present-day reality. At times, I would have to force myself to write down the images that flooded my heart. At the same time, I needed to be husband and father, and my patients needed my thoughtfulness and care. I do not think that I let anyone down. Writing the book has brought me closer to a sense of acceptance, but I am not yet at peace.

What do I now think about my profession? This book must not be viewed as an indictment of psychiatry. There are too many men and women who daily and effectively treat those whose lives have been ravaged by mental illness. There are researchers in the field whose creativity, skill, and ethical responsibility have considerably advanced our understanding of the biological and social factors that contribute to the onset of depression, psychosis, and disorders of various kinds.

This book is an indictment of one psychiatrist. It is an indictment of a government agency gone awry. It is a tale of two national governments that hide behind secrecy and the legal system. I feel good about what I do; I do not blame psychiatry. My search for understanding has at least allowed me to make that distinction and to value without reservation my identity as a physician and as a member of my profession. It is my earnest hope that never again will we see the abuse of human rights that was perpetrated at the Allan Memorial in the name of science.

Yet lurking still are the images of the past. They, too, are part of who I am, and they will remain with me for the rest of my life.

I remember my room when I was fourteen. The walls and carpet were blue; my room looked out on the lawn and garden; the bedspread and curtains, a blue plaid. It had always been a place for me to play, to study, to listen to music. Over the next several years, it became a refuge and then a prison. My heart aches as I remember my father stumbling down the steps or shuffling in the corridor . . . with tears, I remember.

Part 4: The Aftermath

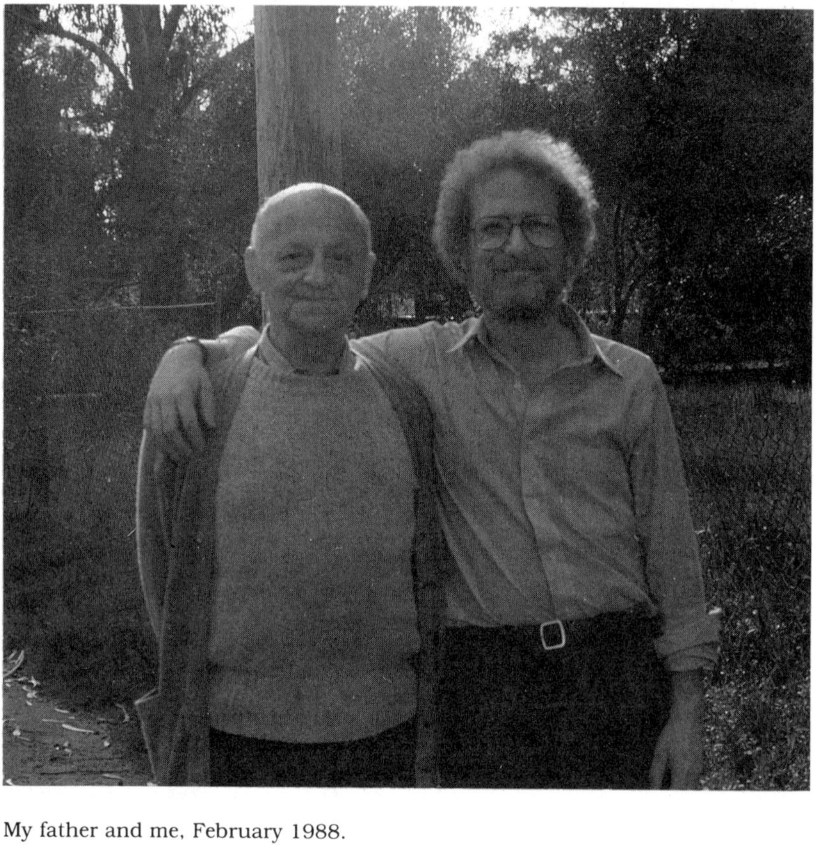

My father and me, February 1988.

Afterword

The Settlement

On October 5, 1988, the *San Francisco Chronicle* front page headline read, "U.S. Settles Suit Over CIA's 'Brainwashing.' " My son, retrieving the paper from the cool early morning dew, raced through the house shouting, his exuberance in stark contrast to the exhaustion felt by his parents. For the first time, I truly knew the story behind the headlines; for the first time as well, I understood how victory can be bittersweet.

The pace had quickened in late spring when Judge Penn reset the the trial date to October 4, 1988. The CIA attorneys, acknowledging the reality that the case would not be thrown out on technical grounds, began in earnest to prepare for trial. Having exhausted all delaying tactics, they demanded the current medical records on each of the plaintiffs. Additionally, they began a search for new expert witnesses and hired several with enviable reputations in medical ethics, the history of psychiatry, and forensic psychiatry. These included Tom Beauchamp, Senior Research Scholar, Center for Bioethics, Kennedy Institute of Ethics, Georgetown University; Eliot Valenstein, Professor of Psychology at the University of Michigan; and Jonas Rappaport, Professor of Psychiatry at the University of Maryland. Present at several of the depositions as an advisor to the government was Park Elliot Dietz, who at that time was Professor of Psychiatry at the University of Virginia and a long-time advisor to the government in issues of psychiatry and law. For the plaintiffs, an equally impressive group of witnesses was arrayed. Included were Robert Jay Lifton, Distinguished Professor of Psychiatry and Psychology at the City University of New York; Leon Salzman, Professor of Psychiatry at Georgetown University Medical School; David J. Rothman, Bernard Schoenberg Professor of Social Medicine and Director, Center for the Study of Society and Medicine, College of Physicians and Surgeons, Columbia University; Omond Solandt, former Chairman of the Canadian Defense Research Board; Alice Olson, widow of Frank Olson; and others. Clearly, the number of eminent witnesses on both sides was beginning to mount, as were the pages of depositions.

The areas of conflict were delineated ever more clearly. Was Cameron's work a deviation in the history of psychiatry? Would he have been expected to inform his patients of the nature of the experiments in any way other than with the customary consent form? Was there proof that the eight Canadians had suffered any permanent damage from Cameron's experiments?

In order to determine the cause and nature of impairment, the CIA attorneys began a review of both the past and current medical records of each of the plaintiffs. Additionally, each would undergo an evaluation by Jonas Rappaport in order to determine their current mental state. As the increasing involvement of the Canadian plaintiffs became a reality, my father's anxiety began to mount. He began to check for the mail many times a day; he would sit by the telephone waiting to hear from Turner or someone else associated with the case; he could talk of nothing else. His sleep became more disturbed as he lay awake for hours musing on what he remembered of the past. As well, he began to obsess about his deposition, going over what he had said again and again, increasingly disturbed about whether he had said the "right thing." His physical complaints began to increase, and my family began to wonder if he would survive this increasingly intense experience.

In the early summer, my father was visited by a social

worker from the University of Virginia who was collaborating with Dr. Rappaport. The interviews were to be conducted without any family member present, and so my sister Terri waited in another room despite my father's wish to have her present for support. In addition, the interview was taped without the permission of the attorneys. The storm of protest that this produced made my father even more upset. As he thought about what he had said, his anxiety became so great that he began to worry about the reaction of the social worker to him. After the interview ended, my father commented to my sister that the woman wore a blouse that was quite low-cut; he felt that she was interested in him. To my great surprise, he also indicated that she had suggested that they have lunch together, and he had invited her to join him at his beloved Montefiore Club. I was puzzled; was this some sort of ploy to see his reactions, or was this a misinterpretation on his part? It was certainly most unusual. His fantasy of what all this meant grew dramatically as he built this into a scene of seduction. After innumerable telephone calls and attempts to learn what had actually transpired, my father canceled plans for any follow-up lunch. The sequence of events was filled with a great deal of emotion on the part of my father, my sister, myself, attorneys, and others. Although the truth is murky, it is possible that in an attempt to master his anxiety, he had turned a threatening situation into one of familiarity. I became concerned about the implication of such unusual behavior. If his response to an interview was so profound, what indeed would happen when he was put on the stand in a courtroom in Washington? I began to ask myself really for the first time, whether he would survive a trial.

I spent most of July reviewing all of my father's current medical records and preparing for my second deposition, which was scheduled for mid-summer. The first deposition had been so grueling and unpleasant that I was not at all looking forward to further interaction with the Justice Department attorney who was handling the case. I was determined, however, to anticipate the line of questioning, and so I reviewed my father's records, old and new, and studied the clinical issues of organic brain syndromes and electroconvulsive treatment. Interspersed in all of this, I read books on the history of psychiatry and psychiatric treatment. In retrospect, I wonder how I managed to keep the many aspects of my life in place, but I was driven by the sense that we were in the home stretch. It was now or never, and we all had come too far to give anything up.

It would be much too simplistic to suggest that this process was not wearing or that it did not at times tear away at my soul. Trying to meet all of my obligations, preparing to be an expert witness, supporting my father, being the spokesperson for my family, and at the same time being a husband and father was grueling. The summer of 1988 was filled with days of dizzying tension as all of the pieces came together prior to trial.

I was plagued as well by another significant source of concern. I had an overriding fear that Jim Turner would not be able to continue if the case were continued very much longer. Nine years earlier, the case had been taken on by Joe Rauh, who had involved his young associate. A reorganization of the firm had resulted in Turner becoming a partner, and within two years, Rauh retired. The costs of a lawsuit against the government of the United States can be enormous, especially when the Justice Department uses tactics that are designed to stonewall, rather than to advance the cause of justice. Since the attorneys were to be paid on a contingency basis, no monies were forthcoming from the plaintiffs, most of whom were impoverished. A small law firm can only carry this kind of burden for a limited period of time. Over the years, we had attempted to raise funds with a campaign across Canada that was organized by Dave Orlikow. Despite the well-known Canadians who lent their names to the fund-raising, only a few thousand dollars were raised. Even the Canadian celebrities who were generous with their names were not forthcoming with their pocketbooks. Resistance came in the form of comments such as, "Why should I give money to pay the lawyers? They will get their due if they win." or "Cameron's patients will get their money when they win. Why should I give any now?" What most did not realize was that, although the initial lawsuit had been for $1,000,000 per plaintiff, Rauh and Turner had very early on offered to settle for $250,000, and when the Canadian government (mistakenly, as it turned out) indicated that the United States government was interested in a settlement in late 1984, they reduced the amount to $175,000.

By 1988, hundreds of thousands of dollars had been charged to time spent by the attorneys, and thousands more were direct out-of-pocket expenses. I wrote letters to friends and family, asking for contributions to the fund. Some money came in, but the total was about $10,000—a drop of water in the vast ocean of government resources. It was clear to me that Jim Turner could not devote the prime of his career to fighting a case with little financial support. Since his energies were devoted to this endeavor, he could only take on a minimal amount of other work, and so his billings for the firm would be low. Could a small law firm continue to carry this expense for the foreseeable future? It remained a puzzle to me how a lawsuit that captured the interest of people across Canada could not capture their generosity.

I must admit that, over the time that we tried to raise funds, I learned a great deal about how negatively lawyers are viewed; the stereotypes coupled with a generalized disinterest made fundraising a joyless proposition. The implications for successful resolution were ominous.

Two different institutions were instrumental in assisting in the financial aspects of the situation. The first was the J. Roderick MacArthur Foundation, which on two occasions granted thousands of dollars to assist in trial preparation. The second was the Mental Health Law Project, a public interest law firm in Washington, D.C., that provides legal services in the arena of patient rights. It was their Director of Litigation, Leonard Rubenstein, who joined Jim Turner as co-counsel to help take the case to its conclusion. It is another of the sad ironies of this story that American citizens and foundations gave of their time and money for nine Canadians while few Canadian citizens and no foundations stepped forward when funds were needed to keep the case alive.

Some months earlier, I had come to Washington to work with the attorneys, and Jim Turner set up a meeting for me to meet with Len Rubenstein. By then, Rauh, Lichtman, Levy & Turner had become Lichtman, Trister & Levy and was ensconced in a suite above Dupont Circle that was considerably more elegant than Joe Rauh's unprepossessing den. We met in a conference room around a large table; legal books filled the bookshelves on all sides. I did not know what to expect. What I found in Len Rubenstein was a lawyer whose humanity and caring shone like a beacon, whose sense of fairness and decency provided an injection of hope at a time that the rest of us (especially Jim) were worn out and on edge from the ups and downs of seven years of fight. Len became my friend.

With funds from these two sources, and with Len assisting Jim for the trial, some of the financial concern was alleviated for the short term. I did not want to think beyond the October trial, but I had serious reservations that if we lost, we would be unable to afford an appeals process.

In August 1988, the second deposition was scheduled, and Len came out to California to be with me during the interrogation. The evening before, Rhona and I went out to dinner with him. It was an unusually balmy evening for Palo Alto, and we ate outside in a garden restaurant. Twinkling lights strung through the branches danced with the light breeze as we sipped wine and ate our meals. My wife Rhona had never met Jim or Joe; she had not previously confronted the reality of the legal process, so Len was the first lawyer with whom she had discussed the case. It was a strange interlude. In a way, it felt like a moment of peace, a chance to reach out to each other as friends; in another way, the discussion made Rhona very much aware that even with the best of preparation, the outcome was uncertain; in addition, the deposition of the following day made me feel as though it were my last dinner. As we talked, however, there was an unmistakable feeling of anticipation. The legal, medical, and psychological issues begged for explication, and in the courtroom history could be made. The feeling of being poised on the brink of a precedent-shattering event filled Rhona and me with excitement. It was an odd moment. The three of us sat there, engulfed by events that we had no part in initiating, buffeted by the winds of the cold war, and by the vagaries of international politics, and the strictures of secrecy.

In the morning, I found myself sitting at another table across from Dan Seikaly, the Justice Department lawyer for the CIA, and the lull was over. It was disconcerting to sit in the conference room of my own department and, yet, to feel that I did not belong there. The process began: the questions, the responses, the explanations. I watched every word, thankful for the training that has made observation a part of my life. To my amazement, something was different this time around. Gone was the adversarial stance; the nasty asides that did not get recorded by the court reporter in the first deposition were gone. The questions were straightforward and exactly what I had expected them to be focused on. But it was the change in demeanor—the sense that, in a subtle way, the theme of the play had been refocused. It was the feeling that the lull of the previous evening had been extended to the battle itself that left me confused. I had put on my armor—I had prepared for the fray—and my enemy offered me cookies. Len provided no explanation, but that was soon forthcoming.

As the weeks passed, and the trial date grew closer, attempts were made to assess economic loss to the plaintiffs. Determining the value of my father's business thirty years prior was not an easy task, but an economist was hired to consult and was able to provide some figures that made possible an assessment of damages. My father had lost hundreds of thousands of dollars of business and work life.

I was sitting at my desk one morning toward the end of August when the telephone rang—it was Jim Turner. He informed me that in July, Joe Rauh had made a personal plea to the new Director of the CIA, William Webster. His letter was masterful and revealed the brilliance of a strategist and the patriotism of a man who believes with all of his heart in the constitution and the civil liberties of the American people. In his letter, which was dated July 20, 1988, he reviewed the numerous attempts made by the attorneys to settle the case, and the refusal to do so by the United States Government lawyers and the CIA. He goes on:

> This direct appeal to you for an appointment comes from a civil libertarian who loves his country and deeply believes it will stand taller at home and throughout the world if it admits past mistakes (with or without admitting legal liability) and provides recompense to those who were injured.
>
> You may wonder why, if plaintiffs' past and present attorneys consider this case so strong, the victims are anxious to settle. I'll tell you why—because they are old and desperate. . . . Their case has already gone on for eight years following an earlier year of fruitless pre-litigation talk. Having observed the protracted delays in even reaching trial (and the recently redoubled government defense with the addition of new lawyers and expert witnesses), I recognize that the road ahead may be a long one, particularly in view of the government's right to appeal to higher courts. Sadly, this litigation could continue until many or most of the remaining victims pass from the scene. This case may well go down in the books as the classic case of "justice delayed, justice denied."

Joe's letter ends with a ringing affirmation of what he has stood for throughout his professional life:

> . . . wouldn't the Agency be a stronger organization by some recognition of error and some recompense therefore? Is it in our nation's interest or tradition to compound the old wrong by continuing the struggle endlessly until many or most of the victims leave this earth with broken lives and without recognition or recompense? A compassionate people can only give one answer.

Joe Rauh may have retired from the practice of law, but he had not lost his interest or energies in pursuing this case to a just conclusion.

Jim's call was my first indication that Joe had indeed written the letter that we had discussed as a possibility at a lunch some time earlier. I now had an explanation for the change in Dan Seikaly's demeanor between the April and August depositions. The CIA finally responded by opening negotiations. Initial discussions hovered around a figure of $250,000 for all plaintiffs or a figure that was not significantly higher than the $25,000 per plaintiff figure that the government had offered some years earlier. Jim finally asked me if I thought that a figure of $500,000 or about $55,000 per plaintiff was acceptable. I was incensed.

"What do you mean?" I sputtered. "You can't be serious! Do you mean that we have worked so hard and fought so long for this measly amount? No, this is not acceptable." There was silence at the other end of the telephone. When Jim spoke, I could tell that he was as angry as I was. "Just because you can help your father financially, I have to think about the others."

I was stunned. I felt attacked, and yet I did not think that this was enough money for anyone. I tried to talk about the idealism that we had all been fighting for, but he countered with a reminder that I was not his client, and that he had to do what was best for his clients. Not his client—true, but I had poured literally years of my life into assisting in preparation of the case. My heart was pounding; I felt betrayed and profoundly disappointed—in Jim and in myself. Finally, he asked me what I would consider acceptable. I could barely respond. My heart was pounding; I felt myself sinking into a well of despair. I struggled to regain my composure and my sense of what I believed in. Finally, I reminded Jim of an earlier meeting, a lunch with Jim, Joe, and Harvey months before in Washington, when Joe had raised that question.

"$100,000 per plaintiff is what we should aim for," I said with resignation, as I reiterated my earlier bottom line. I felt like I had given up. I felt like my father and I had been abandoned, but there seemed to be no choice. There only remained five days before the trial was scheduled to begin, and negotiations had reached a critical phase. Jim also suggested that there might be a maximum amount that the CIA lawyers could negotiate around; a higher figure would require approval at a different level of government. Elliot Lichtman and Jim had immersed themselves in the negotiations, and I knew that the tension was terrible. I was angry, but I felt that I had no right to be. Jim's response made me feel unsure and outraged.

The next day, he called again to tell me that negotiations were continuing. And he apologized. He explained that little sleep, the weight of responsibility, and the passion that he felt for a good and fair resolution had put him on edge. Jim and the others were concerned about what would happen when the plaintiffs took the stand. Would the questioning and the anxiety break them? My comment had felt like an attack on him, and he had fought back. Jim's integrity and single-minded pursuit of justice brought me to my senses, and I remembered how much I owed and respected him. Two stubborn and angry men had to acknowledge the stress of the process and move on—and so we did.

Rhona and I slept poorly on Friday night, September 30. The trial was scheduled to begin on Tuesday, and negotiations were continuing. I had been scheduled to begin testimony the next week, and I was caught between studying and reviewing my notes for the trial and praying for a resolution that would end this tension. We had debated for hours whether we really wanted a settlement. The advantage of a trial was that the issues would be exposed to public scrutiny for weeks. Dirty linen would be aired and the world would see that the story was not only accurate as had been reported, but even worse than had been revealed. Didn't the larger issues cry out for exposure? I knew that a settlement would lead to two to three days of discussion and then oblivion. A trial would sustain the interest. What were the goals, and whose goals were most important?

On Saturday, after Rhona and I had argued about the best course of action, I called Len Rubenstein. Len expressed the ambivalence that I had been wrestling with for twenty-four hours; he too was torn. He reviewed the negotiations, he described how the strategy was evolving, he confirmed the pressure that Jim and Elliot were working under, and he described a strategy lunch with Joe Rauh. He reminded both of us that it was not a certainty that we would win, and we had to consider that as a possibility. When he described how the other plaintiffs were faring under the pressure, I recognized how my concern had been raised when my father reacted so badly to the psychiatric evaluation. He then helped us to frame the goal that we had been searching for all night; the objective of all of this was to ensure that nine Canadian citizens who had been victimized by the CIA would not only receive an acknowledgment that their lives counted for something, but that in their lifetimes, money would be available to ease their situations. Our concerns about intelligence secrecy, the misuse of innocent citizens—all that was important but not at the expense of achieving restitution for those who had suffered. And so, we acquiesced; no, we embraced the position, and we waited for the final negotiations.

On Sunday, Jim called to check in again, faithfully keeping me abreast of all that was taking place three thousand miles away. He had spent much of the weekend speaking with all of the plaintiffs and making certain that he had their go-ahead before accepting any settlement offer. That evening, Dave Orlikow called. He and Val had been debating the same issues that Rhona and I were pursuing. He too arrived at the same conclusion and felt pretty confident in the decision. He told me that Val wanted to talk with me. Over the years, I have grown very fond of Val Orlikow, but I was not at all sure that I wanted to talk with her then. If she had strongly negative opinions, I was going to hear them. And I did. Val felt strongly that the settlement was insufficient, that an apology from the CIA was essential, and that we should hold out. We talked for a long time, neither convincing the other, and yet, when the conversation ended, I knew that she too would embrace the strategy as the most reasonable approach.

Over the weekend, the hours dragged by. I went from one extreme position to the other; I shouted at Rhona; I was irritable with my sons. What kind of payoff would make all the hours of work worthwhile for me? Was I just being selfish? Should I be an idealist who believed that the only good outcome was one in which the system changed? Or should I recognize that the only good solution was one in which the nine victims could feel reinstated as whole human beings? And so, despite my conversation with Len, despite my decision, the ambivalence persisted.

These events all took place in the context of a media blitz. Newspapers prepared to send reporters to Washington to cover what promised to be a sensational exposé of an intelligence service that provokes both powerful feelings and fantasies of bravado. On Saturday, October 1, while we were anxiously awaiting word, the *Toronto Globe and Mail* featured a story by Anne Collins, a Canadian author who had covered the story for several years, titled "Blowing Their Cover: Canadian Victims Take the CIA to Court." The *Chicago Tribune* on Monday, October 3, "Canadians Test CIA Over Brainwashing"; the *London Sunday Telegraph*, September 25, "Brainwashing Challenge to CIA"; and the *Southam News*, "Stakes Are High as Brainwash Case Gets Day in Court." On Monday, October 3, Michael Taylor of the *San Francisco Chronicle* published a piece that he had begun the week before, titled "Trial for CIA Brainwashing Case." On the Saturday night that Rhona and I were tensely awaiting a call from Len Rubenstein, I participated in a long interview with the Stanford University News and Publications Office. I could not let on to anyone that negotiations were proceeding, so my interviews were exceedingly uncomfortable as I played the role of anticipating a difficult trial.

When Jim and I had first spoken the previous week, I telephoned my father to see what made sense to him. I discussed the fact that the two sides were in discussion and asked him if there was an amount of money that would allow him to feel some recompense. "Well, sonny-boy, I have to think about that." He was silent for a long time. "What figure did you say they started with?" "A quarter of a million," I said. "That doesn't give me very much, does it?" "No, Dad." Silence. "Did Mr. Turner have anything else to say?" "No, Dad." "Well, I would say that if I could have $100,000. . . ." He started to sob and had trouble finishing the sentence. "All right, Dad, $100,000 it is." He choked, and said abruptly, "I'll speak with you later, son."

On Sunday, he called to ask if I had heard any more. My sisters called, and we waited.

On Monday, October 3, I had just completed a radio interview for the Canadian Broadcasting Association when I received a call from Jim. He was exhilarated and his voice sounded several octaves higher than usual. "We got it! $750,000 for the plaintiffs. That will work out to $100,000 in Canadian funds for each one." I felt teary; I wanted to rise out of my seat and yell at the top of my lungs, and at the same time I was weighed down by a feeling of intense emptiness and despair. It was not the amount of money that troubled me; it was the realization that even in victory, the memories would never be erased. Was justice possible when life was experienced in a shadow? Superimposed on this was the recognition that the moment was ended; an opportunity to influence government and professional awareness had passed. I went with the first feeling and thanked Jim for all that he and Joe had done; I very sincerely praised his intellect and perseverance. Without these men, there would only have been the web of helplessness ensnaring the victims and their families in a never-ending trap of depression and paralysis. Jim explained that the amount required approval from the Attorney General's office, but he expected that to be pro forma.

I waited a minute and caught my breath as I looked out the office window. I felt dazed, almost unbelieving that it was over. A kaleidoscope of images flashed through my mind as I thought about Mrs. Huard, Mr. Page, Dr. Morrow, and the others. We had come to the end of the road. The leaves were golden against the California-blue sky, and a young woman, jogging by, stopped to rest against a tree beside the building. She saw me and waved, full of life, full of the boundless enthusiasm for confronting the world that is so manifest in Stanford students; her smile brought me to earth and I quickly called my dad.

"It's over. You got what you wanted. The final settlement is $750,000 American. Isn't that great?" "Yes . . . son. . . ." His tears started and then I joined him. I wished that we were in the same room so that I could hold him. For once, my ambivalence was gone. I could only feel love and sorrow for all that he had lost. In that moment, we were bound closer than we had ever been, and would ever be. Even then, even in that moment of such intimacy, the longing for my mother emerged. "I wish Mom could have been here." He cried anew. Finally I said good-bye, to face the barrage of telephone calls that began as soon as I put the receiver down.

The Aftermath

The settlement announcement on Tuesday, October 5, 1988, was cautiously interpreted by government attorneys as tentative and requiring further approval. Turner commented, however, at that point, "This is a statement that every part of our government is under the law. . . ." The response of the CIA through its spokesman, Bill Devine, was quite illustrative, "Any settlement, if approved, does not represent a concession of liability on the part of the agency."

Controversy continued at the time of settlement. Val Orlikow, initially angry and disappointed, was quoted in the media as saying that the CIA had merely "flicked a flea off the sleeve of their jacket. . . . I know that the CIA has blinked and that blink is better than nothing." This comment was interpreted by some as evidence that the attorneys might have acted without full consent of all the plaintiffs, but as Jim Turner pointed out, "I had an unambiguous and airtight authorization to go forward with this [settlement] from every one of my clients." True, I had mixed feelings and so had the Orlikows, but clearly there was only one choice. Settlement means compromise, and compromise means that something is given up by both parties. For us it was the opportunity to fight in a public arena; for the CIA, they awarded the largest amount of money ever given to foreign citizens by the United States as the result of a lawsuit and the largest award ever given by the CIA. Shortly thereafter, Val Orlikow and her daughter flew to Washington, D.C., to thank the attorneys and to take them all out for a dinner of celebration.

During the next week, I gave over a hundred interviews—radio call-in shows, television talk shows, and newspapers from all over the United States and Canada. From morning to night, I performed, trying to explain why we settled, what the settlement meant, how my father had responded. It was then that I began to gain an inkling that others saw the settlement in a different light. "How could you settle for so little? Dr. Weinstein, don't you think that the CIA got off scot-free?" Canadians felt as though they had been sold out to the United States; many American reporters were shocked that they had never heard of the case until this point, despite all of our attempts at raising interest over the years. The response in the print media ranged from jubilant to sarcastic.

The Washington Post; October 6, 1988:

> Subjects of CIA Mind Control View Settlement as a Victory

Chicago Tribune, October 5, 1989:

> CIA Brainwashing Suit Settled

U.S. News and World Report, October 17, 1988:

> A Cold-War Horror Show's Last Act

Vancouver Sun, October 5, 1988:

> Payout Brings End to Struggle

The Washington Post, October 18, 1988:

> . . . it is a very real expression of this country's regret and acceptance of responsibility. It is, and has been for eight years, the only decent and honorable conclusion to this episode.

And then other perspectives began to appear.

From an editorial in the *Toronto Star*, shortly after the settlement:

> . . . how can there be a full sense of justice if the CIA offers cash, but refuses to apologize for the outrages committed on unsuspecting Canadians?. . . A full sense of justice for the Canadian victims will also not be achieved as long as the Canadian government—the major funder of the clinic conducting the experiments—makes public the complicity of the government of the day. The CIA's settlement certainly represents a strong statement of culpability. Sadly, it still falls short of a full apology.

From the *Vancouver Courier*, October 9, 1989, a cartoon by G. Ocson depicts a CIA man in a trenchcoat throwing some pennies at a group of small figures, older men and women with their hands up. The CIA man says: "OK, look. . . .

Sometimes defending the free world means drug experiments on the subjects of other democracies, with their government's assistance. . . . So here's some spare change. . . . NOW GET OFF MY CASE!!" At the lower left corner is a Canadian beaver walking quickly away and saying, "Yeah. . . . Give the guy a break, willya?"

An editorial in the *Montreal Gazette*, October 6, 1988:

> Yet the CIA has won a victory of sorts. For a cost equivalent to the annual salaries of a few minor functionaries, the agency has dodged a formal test of the morality of its actions in open court.

The editorial goes on to castigate the Government of Canada:

> Having salved its conscience with a paltry $20,000 payment to each of its victims earlier this year, Ottawa continues to evade the more profound questions. How does a state based on concepts of natural justice and rooted in the rule of law, a state which claims to protect its citizens—how does such a state come to persuade itself that tormenting its most helpless is in the interests of national security? The U.S. government and its creature, the CIA, may have avoided grappling with such questions. Canada should not. If the stain cannot be erased, the government can at least take ownership of its sin. That is how a true democracy protects itself.

And finally, a letter appeared in the *Montreal Gazette* during the week after the settlement. Its headline read, "Was Doctor Victim, Too?" Once again, the writer uses the label of "psychiatric patients" to diminish the claim of the nine victims and to proclaim the best intentions of Ewen Cameron.

The differing perspectives that these news articles represent were to surface repeatedly over the next months as I talked with many who followed the case to its conclusion.

Rhona, our sons, and I had been scheduled to visit Washington for the trial beginning the week of October 10. Despite the settlement, we decided to go anyway, so that we could thank those whose work had made a good outcome possible. In multiple rounds of celebration, we heard the message repeatedly that the settlement was a significant victory. I felt elated. I felt vindicated. I felt proud.

That same week, the Canadian edition of this book was published with the title *A Father, A Son, and the CIA*. Fortuitously, the settlement of the case had coincided with the release of the story, and I was scheduled to begin a cross-Canada publicity tour immediately after leaving Washington. During the following eight days, my balloon of joy was punctured repeatedly by charges that we had sold out and by comments that I had not stood up to my profession. Despite words of support from some in the news media, others wounded with attacks on the integrity of the lawyers and on my own motivations. During the book tour, I was exposed to the dichotomous responses at first hand. Within one week, I became aware that, as I suspected, interest would rapidly wane—the lessons lost.

Although the book was warmly received by most, it was dismissed by others as too emotional, a sob-story or another story about a mental patient; it was described by one reviewer as a book along the lines of "the CIA-made-my-father-sick." The same reviewer goes on:

> That editorial reviewers across the country shiver with indignation about the CIA ruining Canadian lives with its wicked experiments shows just how vulnerable we still are to schoolboy conspiracy theories. I mean, really. It's just like living in Iran and hearing daily about the "Great Satan."

Once again, to my great distress, comments designed to diminish the extent of duplicity and tragedy were published by someone who had no intimate knowledge of the case. This review was written especially for the *Montreal Gazette*, a paper that had closely followed the case for nine years. My letter to the editor in response was neither published nor acknowledged. Despite multiple positive reviews elsewhere, it was this one that indicated how the overall response to settlement would turn out, for Canadians would soon choose to forget. The Government of Canada would be released by its own citizens from responsibility for its actions both in funding the experiments and in supporting the CIA in the protracted lawsuit.

Complacency—the Canadian way of life. With the assistance of Linda Hunt, an investigative journalist in Washington, I had obtained a list of ten Canadians who had attended meetings of the Tripartite Commission at Edgewood Army Arsenal in Maryland in 1954. These meetings were set up by the American, Canadian, and British to review and discuss chemical and biological warfare methods during the time that the American military, the CIA, and the Canadian defense establishment were focused on mind control as a major concern. I was unable to obtain from the Canadian Government any information about these men or the meetings under the Access to Information Act. The reply was that release of such data required the permission of the United States and would not be given—even though I had asked about the positions and roles of these scientists in Canada. I heard from National Defense two months after the case had been settled and decided to pass the information on to some Canadian group that might be interested in investigating it further. I therefore sent the information to the *Toronto Globe and Mail*, one of the newspapers that had castigated the Government of Canada for its role in funding Ewen Cameron over the years. I received no acknowledgment.

In the United States, there were a few stories that appeared over the next month. On October 26, 1988, the *Stanford Campus Report* published an opinion piece by two scientists, Michael Wrona and Mark Branagh, calling on their brethren to heed my concern that the issues raised by MKULTRA and the Tuskegee experiments should continue to be debated and examined by scientists and academicians:

> Who, if not a community of scholars, is in a position to initiate and direct the dialogue necessary to understand the ramifications of such acts?
>
> It is time for those of us who can fathom the ramifications of such misdirected applications of science and medicine to make our collective voices heard. We must promote open dis-

course about MKULTRA and similar programs. We must understand, and make others understand—before it's too late to learn from our mistakes.

Len Rubenstein published a piece in *The New York Times* on November 7, 1988, that concludes, "Let us be wary then, not just of CIA abuses but of ambitious yet misguided experiments performed in the name of treatment." I talked to a few groups, including the Technology and Society Committee of Silicon Valley and the Santa Clara County Democratic Coalition, and appeared on a few more television shows. The interest, however, was sporadic. My greatest fears had come to pass—settlement was tantamount to burial of the issues.

Although I recognized that further public discussion was unlikely, there were still three goals that I felt necessary to fulfill before I personally could put the case to rest. The first was to obtain from the American Psychiatric Association an official statement of regret; the second was to obtain the same from the Canadian Psychiatric Association and the Canadian Medical Association; the third was to lobby the Government of Canada to repudiate the Cooper Report and to make a just payment to the nine victims.

Given the nature of the case, my personal involvement, and the profession that I have chosen, it is not surprising that I had long been distressed by the lack of involvement of the American Psychiatric Association (APA) in any aspect of the process of legal resolution. Early on, I had written to inform the president about the issues, and I asked other colleagues to write as well. As the evidence mounted from 1984 through 1987, I wanted the Association to actively support the case either through a legal brief or by publicity and discussion of the historical, ethical, and moral themes. In 1988, I submitted a proposal for the APA annual meeting, to be held in Montreal, for a panel presentation that would focus on the issues raised by the case. The members of the panel were to be Robert Lifton, M.D., a leader in the study of coercive persuasion and totalitarianism; Jay Katz, M.D., J.D., who is well known in the field of psychiatry and the law and who had written the strong opinion in the Tuskegee case; Margaret Sommerville, Director of the McGill University Center for Medicine, Law, and Ethics; Svend Robinson, member of the Canadian Parliament; and myself. The proposal was rejected, despite my pleadings that not only would it be of intellectual interest, but the timing in Montreal was critical since it would reach the psychiatrists of the two countries. It was suggested that I resubmit it for the following year's meeting in San Francisco. This indicated to me that, perhaps, other issues were involved, such as the need to avoid provoking Canadian psychiatrists. My attempts to put together a panel for the 1989 meeting met with failure, as I could not assemble the same group, nor could I enlist new speakers.

I did not give up, however, in trying to involve the APA in the legal process. I redoubled my efforts and met with Melvin Sabshin, the medical director of the Association, who was compassionate, thoughtful, probing, and clearly aware of the APA's political obligations. He offered research assistance but did not feel that the APA could submit a "friend of the court" brief, nor could it assist with funding. I was aware that within the membership were psychiatrists who had worked with Cameron and who still revered him, but the facts were incontrovertible. Did the Association represent me as well? And who represented the well-being of our patients? At the conclusion of my meeting with the medical director, I felt that there was some question as to whether I was objective about the data and whether I was not viewed as some sort of troublemaker. There was nothing directly put into words, yet I felt that I was being placated. Although disappointed in my colleagues, there was little more that I could do at that point.

Following the settlement, I contacted members of the Northern California Psychiatric Society (NCPS), some of whom had previously written letters to the APA. This society is a district branch of the APA and represents over thirteen hundred psychiatrists in Northern California, more than half the entire number of psychiatrists in Canada. I explained that no branch of our profession or of medicine in general had made any public comment that indicated support of the settlement or concern for what had taken place.

I was invited to address the executive committee within the month. During that time, a letter appeared in *Psychiatric News*, the newspaper of the American Psychiatric Association, confronting psychiatry's responsibility for its past involvement in this matter and its future obligations. It was written by a member of the NCPS whom I had never met. Given the settlement and this further support, the NCPS executive committee voted to release a statement, and I was asked to prepare a first draft. On December 6, 1989, a statement was finally released by Maurice Rappaport, M.D., president of the Society. Included are these words:

> The Northern California Psychiatric Society wishes to express its deepest regret that psychiatric patients became unwitting participants in experimental procedures. Examination of the medical records indicates that no meaningful form of consent was involved. It would also appear that the line between therapy and experimentation was blurred, raising questions of ethical responsibility *even at that time* [emphasis added].
>
> . . . The NCPS encourages physicians to be ever watchful that no further abuses of the civil liberties of our patients be permitted to take place. A physician who becomes aware of such deviation from standard practice has the obligation to ensure that an external review be undertaken.

The NCPS statement articulated two very critical points. First, that Cameron's work was unethical not just with respect to today's procedures, but was in fact unacceptable within the contemporary framework in which Cameron worked. Second, it places responsibility on physicians to break silence when confronted with unethical or questionable practice—a shadow that darkens the Cameron case as well as those of Tuskegee, the Nazi physicians, Russian psychiatry, and Latin American and South African medicine.

The statement was released throughout northern California. It was picked up only by one radio station, one television station, and one newspaper, the *San Francisco Chronicle*, and that only because it was sent directly to Michael Taylor, the reporter who had covered the case in October.

Given the support of the NCPS, I wanted to encourage the

APA to move forward, especially since they were sending a fact-finding team to the Soviet Union to investigate Soviet psychiatry. I wrote to the president of the Association and others asking how the APA could evaluate abuses in other countries if it could not acknowledge the past abuses of American psychiatry. By early spring 1989, the APA Public Affairs Office began to develop a statement that was originally planned to coincide with a press conference relating the experiences of the American psychiatrists who had visited the Soviet Union. The statement was not released at that time. Finally, a decision was made for the statement to be released at the opening press conference of the APA annual meeting in San Francisco in May 1989, eight months after the settlement. The press release, issued by Paul Fink, M.D., who was then president of the American Psychiatric Association, followed the gist of the statement released in December by the NCPS.

> The APA joins our member society in expressing our deep regret that psychiatric patients became unwitting participants in those experiments. . . . In my view, the research . . . could not be conducted today, and *should not have been conducted then*, no matter how frustrated and desperate researchers were to find treatments for those with mental illness [emphasis added].
>
> We as a profession have a responsibility to demand external review when we find or suspect violations of patient protections.

So far as I am aware, this statement by the association representing 35,000 American psychiatrists was reported by only one Canadian newspaper. After the release of the APA statement, I met with Dr. Fink and Dr. Sabshin, the medical director, who encouraged me to submit another symposium for the 1990 meeting of the APA. They were quite supportive, and Dr. Sabshin especially demonstrated his warmth and humanity as he asked about my father. As I thought about a symposium, I felt that the moment had passed. Such a panel discussion would now be lost in the swirl of what was current. Even though I felt the issues to be timeless, I was concerned that they would likely receive little attention in a large meeting without some current provocation. In retrospect, there were two other factors. I had become discouraged the previous year by the lack of interest from some whom I asked to participate in the panel, and I was tired of acting as a one-man conscience for the Association. Preventing the abuse of patients was not my crusade alone. However, by issuing the statement, the APA had finally come through in its own way, and for that I was grateful. There was no question in my mind that if I were going to stand up to the attacks on psychiatry that dogged my steps as I spoke, I needed to feel that my American colleagues had responded. And they did.

On October 8, 1988, the *British Medical Journal* in an editorial took Canadian psychiatry to task for not directly addressing the concerns raised by the case:

> The Canadian psychiatric fraternity has been remarkably coy about the episode. Its psychiatric association has issued a statement. . . . I could not find this statement published in *The Canadian Journal of Psychiatry* up to June 1988. Other Canadian medical journals have been similarly reticent to discuss the many ethical, political, and medical issues raised by this episode. "Why stir things up?" the representative of one asked me recently.

The Canadian Psychiatric Association (CPA) had indeed produced a statement on the issue, although it is still not clear to me where or how it was presented. The statement begins with an affirmation of the importance of the Allan Memorial Institute to Canadian psychiatry. It goes on to note that Cameron applied for grants by following the usual channels and mechanisms of the time and published in peer-reviewed journals. It then closes with a statement of today's policies and concludes that "[s]uch experiments would not be permitted in today's research climate."

Missing in the statement is a sense that there was anything wrong in what Cameron had done; no concern whatsoever was expressed for the patients whose lives were destroyed by "experimentation gone wild with scant criteria," to quote the eminent Canadian psychiatrist, Robert Cleghorn. Missing is an acknowledgment that there is much to be learned, and that misguided protection of one's colleagues and institutions leads only to an erosion of the integrity of the profession.

I received a copy of the statement after I contacted the Canadian Psychiatric Association and forwarded to them a copy of the *British Medical Journal* editorial and the NCPS statement. On March 9, 1989, I received a reply from Dr. Quentin Rae-Grant, Chairman of the Board of Directors of the CPA. His letter reaffirms the statement that was issued and closes as follows: "The Canadian Psychiatric Association, whose view I have just presented above, is not considering further actions or statements with regard to this unfortunate situation." On the same date, I received a letter from Dr. John Bennett, Associate Secretary General of the Canadian Medical Association, that their Executive Committee would be soliciting opinions from "those who are more knowledgeable in the matter raised." I knew at once that this meant input from the Canadian Psychiatric Association, and I further knew what response I would receive.

Indeed, on May 25, 1989, Dr. Bennett wrote as follows:

> It was the committee's view that the CPA's opinion and its statement of June 6, 1987 indicating that the experimentation protocols of thirty years ago as followed by the Allan Memorial Institute in Montreal were, in hindsight, unacceptable by today's standards and would not be followed in today's research, was acceptable to the CMA. The committee recommended that no further action be taken by the CMA in this matter.

He further pointed out that the CMA had in 1975 endorsed the part of the World Medical Association Declaration of Tokyo, which included the statement of condemnation of "the infliction of physical or mental suffering in whatever degree . . . or to cooperate in any other way unwillingly." So, on the one hand, the CMA supported a condemnation of misuse of patients around the world; on the other, it would not condemn experimentation carried out thirty years earlier in its own backyard, nor would it express any regret for the abuse of unwitting patients. The British Medical Association termed the actions of the CPA "coy." I saw the actions of the CPA and the CMA as cowardice. I brought these responses to the attention of the Canadian media—once again, to no avail. There was nothing more that I could do.

The final task that I set out for myself was to ascertain whether the Government of Canada could be persuaded to assume the responsibility it had cast aside with the Cooper Report. On December 14, 1988, I wrote the Minister of Justice, enclosing copies of the NCPS statement and the editorial from the *British Medical Journal*:

> Both of these statements suggest, Mr. Minister, that physicians around the world do not excuse the actions of Ewen Cameron as did the so-called expert witnesses (Grunberg, Lowy, and McDonald) in their reports for the Cooper Opinion. Furthermore, they are an indication that many do not see how Canadian medicine and the Government of Canada can sidestep responsibility on the basis of the Cooper Opinion. During an era when there is major concern about human rights and medical torture supported by totalitarian regimes world-wide, one could hope that an enlightened Canadian government would directly face its own responsibility for past violations.

I asked in the letter that the Government of Canada make an *ex gratia* payment to the plaintiffs that would be commensurate with the pain and suffering that each had experienced. I asked further that the government follow the suggestion of Mr. Cooper, and rectify the demeaning message that the earlier payment had sent. On March 7, 1989, I received a letter from Doug Lewis, the Minister of Justice and Attorney General of Canada. The final paragraph of his letter sums up the response of a government that bought its way out of a predicament at minimal cost; a government that did not have the courage to face its own mistakes.

> The Government of Canada supported the objective of an early resolution to the lawsuit against the United States Govern-

> ment which has now been resolved. The Canadian government has provided assistance, including funding of legal expenses on an ex gratia basis, to nine former patients who sued the Government of the United States. Having examined its own involvement in funding medical research, the Government of Canada does not consider that a payment on its part is warranted.

Since with few exceptions, there had never been strong support among members of parliament for fighting this case, and since public response indicated a desire to bury the issues, I had no recourse at that point but to give up.

We had won in the settlement. I had lost within my own profession in Canada; I had lost with the government of the country of my birth; and, most of all, I had lost because the ethical, moral, and professional issues were relegated to yesterday's headlines. One year later, I am aware that mixed with the feelings of elation lie feelings of anger. The core of helplessness that haunted me through the years remains barely touched by the lawsuit that was to demolish its pernicious presence. And so, the victory was bittersweet, and we await the lessons of history to see if anything was learned.

Reflections

"I can't stand your pain," she said, softly.

The moment will remain with me for a very long time. The therapeutic mask had been stripped away; the professional persona evaporated with her words. During the months that I was working on this book, I had often wondered how its publication and the media coverage of the lawsuit would affect my patients. Some handled the revelations with a kind of vicarious pride; others grappled with the experience of knowing more about a therapist than they had ever wanted. Therapy hours became focused on me as activist or me as victim. Alternating themes of helplessness and the quest for control pervaded the treatment process as we tried to deal with the reality of my life superimposed on a fantasied reality of who they thought I was. In each situation, it became the focus of the work for months. Ultimately, I am satisfied that, for most of my patients, the therapeutic outcome has been positive, but I am left with a question. Where is the line? When does biography become a dangerous endeavor? The forces that propelled me to write this book were the most powerful that I have ever experienced. Certainly I realized that writing this book could have profound implications for my patients who knew me in another way. And yet, I do not believe that I broke their trust. I believe the affirmation that strength can grow out of weakness; that I too am a man who has struggled; that these facets of my past provided a framework on which we could build a healing process.

From this experience with my patients, however, I have taken away a strong lesson. Once again, I am reminded of the power of physicians, of the power of the therapeutic encounter, and of the trust that our patients place in us—a trust that we must not break.

As I have talked with interested people throughout the United States and Canada, one question recurs. Is MKULTRA or its equivalent happening now? Could it happen again?

I do not know if such experiments are surreptitiously part of the fabric of our society today. What frightens me and gives me pause, however, is that the structures which supported the work of Ewen Cameron and the other physicians, psychologists, and researchers still exist. This is most clear in the inability of Canadian medicine and psychiatry to acknowledge a past transgression. It is further apparent in the resistance of both the American and Canadian governments to acknowledge responsibility for their misuse of innocent citizens. It is painfully apparent in the silence of those who have heard the evidence and do not respond.

Why do I believe this danger to be with us still despite the evolution of human subjects committees and peer review mechanisms? My concern lies both in the structure of medicine as a profession and in what history has taught us about human nature. Within the Hippocratic oath lies the following promise: "To hold my teacher in this art equal to my parents."

If, in fact, this oath reflects a philosophy of medical education and training that is active today, then the implication is worrisome. Although we learn to question the judgments of our parents, it is quite clear that for a critical period in our development their guidance is paramount. Even at later points in our lives, however, their voices can influence and determine our behaviors, at times even when we might choose a different path. Certainly, medicine has evolved to a point where we recognize that our heroes may have feet of clay, but medicine has been a fairly authoritarian profession. There has been a historical tendency within the field to elevate the teachers and researchers, and to attribute to them a breadth of wisdom and integrity that may not always be deserved. The corollary is that "lesser" colleagues may hold back, and disagreement may be stifled. It may be that one reason for the significant involvement of philosophers, theologians, and other nonmedical scholars in the study of bioethics is the concern that medical professionals cannot move beyond this traditional paternalistic model. How else can we explain the reluctance of the Canadian Psychiatric Association to repudiate the work of an eminent psychiatrist? How else can I understand the response of a well-known American psychiatrist, when I wrote to enlist his assistance in the CIA case, that Cameron was a great teacher and that he could not say anything negative about him?

An examination of the Cameron case as well as a consideration of the rise and fall of German medicine in this century provides useful but frightening data about the weak underbelly of a worthy profession. Alexander Capron in a review of the history of German medicine makes the frightening point that German medicine had developed stringent directives against the misuse of patients by 1900, and these were further developed by the 1930s. He notes that in 1900, the Prussian government issued a policy statement to the heads of medical clinics that "prohibited medical interventions for purposes other than diagnosis, therapy, or immunization" under the following conditions: if the patient were a minor or not fully competent, if there were no clear and unambiguous consent, and if that consent was given only after all possible consequences were described. This directive was striking and innovative because it protected vulnerable patients, it required disclosure, and it placed the onus of responsibility on the directors of the medical institutions. By 1931, German medicine had regulations concerning such issues as therapeutic and human experimentation. But less than a decade later, that same enlightened body was carrying out experimentation on incarcerated and helpless men, women, and children under the policies and direction of the Third Reich.

It is the silence and resistance to truth that makes us all vulnerable. I am haunted by the silence of my colleagues who worked at the Allan Memorial Institute in the 1950s and did not speak up; I am appalled by their continued silence in the 1980s when the truth emerged. Medicine has a history of engaging in evil undertakings when the motivation can be reframed so that the outcome is couched under the rubric of "for the greater good." The nontreatment of syphilis by the United States Public Health Service, the experimentation of the Nazi doctors for the good of the Fatherland, the irresponsible destruction of psychiatric patients under the guise of "curing their schizophrenia"—all of these found willing adherents, physicians who would carry out the work for a larger philosophy of good intention. Phillip Zimbardo, a social psychologist at Stanford University, terms this phenomenon the "structure of evil." The actors engage in evil for a "good" reason.

Even more disturbing, however, is the process under which reasonable, educated men and women can assume this motivation. The second factor is the presence of a charismatic leader, one who has the power to promote and the power to withhold. Cameron was such a man. By establishing himself as the leader, being granted the allegiance of his students as enshrined in the philosophy of the Hippocratic oath, and being given significant power to build the careers of his followers, he could frame his ambitions in terms of "healing schizophrenia" and build a structure capable of destroying human minds in a zeal to cure. It was not Ewen Cameron who pushed the buttons daily; it was not Cameron who spent the day nursing the disoriented patients in the sleep rooms. Those tasks were carried out by the functionaries of his empire.

Medicine continues to be a vulnerable profession. Its philosophical bent is toward granting significant power to its teachers; its structures promote cure and the greater good—a perspective that if not always questioned may lead us to act in ways that may not be in the best interests of our patients. Despite the consumer movement and the influence of regulatory bodies, patienthood is still a role assumed by adults in which power is given up over one's own body. Usually, this is done in an atmosphere of trust and with an expectation that the patient and therapist share a common goal. As we have seen time and again throughout the history of medicine, that assumption does not always follow.

I have been criticized by some for not blaming psychiatry and medicine for participating in the work of the CIA. I still believe that my profession is a noble calling, but as the months have passed, my concerns about an inherent weakness, a point of potential rupture in the steel of good intentions, lead me to encourage my colleagues to learn from our mistakes. How can we be afraid to heal ourselves?

And so, forty years later, by avoiding the past, the medical establishment continues to condone the goals and policies of Cameron. By the silence of his colleagues and by the inability of medicine's professional bodies to confront a transgression, the leader stands unchallenged—his work considered acceptable because it was carried out in an attempt to find a cure for one of the greatest human ills. If we have learned nothing from the experiments in Montreal, if we have learned nothing from the deaths of those who died in MKULTRA or related experiments, then we are all at risk and, despite the work of human subjects committees and institutional review boards, we will all be vulnerable.

One year later—it is autumn 1989, and the protagonists of this drama have moved on.

Jim Turner continues to practice law in Washington, D.C., and has moved to another law firm.

Joe Rauh enjoys his retirement with the ebullience and energy that characterized his career.

Len Rubenstein takes on new cases testing the bounds of mental health law in this country.

David Orlikow lost his seat in the House of Commons during the election of autumn 1988. After 26 years, the NDP Member of Parliament had lost his first election in 18 consecutive tries at elected office. An era was ended. How the CIA suit influenced this outcome is not clear, but the election was held one month after the settlement. Canada lost a parliamentarian whose commitment to human rights was a model to all.

Svend Robinson fought one of the most bitter campaigns ever for his seat in the House of Commons. Before the election, he revealed his homosexuality, which then became a focus of the campaign. Brian Mulroney disgraced himself by what appeared to be blatant homophobic comments. Svend won reelection with a significant majority.

Val Orlikow remains in Winnipeg, trying to put the lives of her family back together.

Robert Logie used some of his money to buy a condominium in Vancouver. He finally has some security. Logie is trying to mount a new fight against the Government of Canada.

Jean Charles Page moved from the barely livable house that he had occupied to a new place in Ontario, ready to start again.

Mary Morrow, whom we felt should share in the settlement, has more money to put into a comfortable retirement.

Jeanine Huard, too, has a degree of security that was beyond her grasp. She has a job as a caregiver of the elderly and lives in a small apartment in the north end of Montreal.

My father, Lou Weinstein, has changed his life very little. He took a vacation in Florida with friends, and he delights in his family. He continues to fight the mood swings and memories. A lawsuit filed several years ago against the Royal Victoria Hospital moves slowly toward a conclusion.

I do not know about the rest of the plaintiffs.

Brian Mulroney won reelection as Prime Minister of Canada.

Joe Clark won reelection and continues as External Affairs Minister.

Raymond Hnatyshyn lost his seat in Parliament and was recently named Governor General of Canada.

George Schultz is back at Stanford as an esteemed professor in the School of Business.

As for me, I have been changed for the better in ways that are subtle yet distinct. I have a greater awareness of those who have been abused; I am not afraid to fight for my beliefs. But when asked, Was all of this a catharsis? Did the settlement and writing the book end the sadness? my answer is simple: I reached for the brass ring; for a moment, I held it and savored the joy. And then, it was out of my grasp. My fingers still feel the solidity of resolution, but my heart feels the emptiness of dashed hopes.

In November 1988, the United States Senate approved legislation to establish an Inspector General for the CIA independent of the CIA's director. This individual would be nominated by the president and approved by the Senate. This arrangement will permit a more thorough investigation of any wrongdoing committed by the Agency.

Sources

Prologue

Marks, John. *The Search for the Manchurian Candidate: The CIA and Mind Control.* New York: Times Books, 1979.

Chapter 7

Braceland, Francis J. "In memorium. D. Ewen Cameron, 1901–1967." *American Journal of Psychiatry* 124:860–861, 1967.

Cleghorn, R.A. "The emergence of psychiatry at McGill." *Canadian Journal of Psychiatry* 29:551–556, 1982.

Zilboorg, Gregory. "Biographical sketch, D. Ewen Cameron, President, 1952–53." *American Journal of Psychiatry* 110:10–12, 1953.

Several of the reported interviews were carried out by Jay Peterzell of the Center for National Security Studies in preparation for John Marks's book, *The Search for the Manchurian Candidate*. In the intervening years, publicity and lawsuits have made many of Cameron's colleagues less willing to discuss these issues.

Cameron, D. Ewen. "General thoughts about my years as Director of the Institute." From *Medical Institutes*, unpublished manuscript in the Archives of the American Psychiatric Association, Washington, D.C.

Cameron, D. Ewen. Letter to F. Cyril James, Principal Emeritus of McGill University, March 14, 1964. Archives of the American Psychiatric Association, Washington, D.C.

Cameron, D. Ewen. *Objective and Experimental Psychiatry*, New York: The MacMillan Company, 1941.

Cameron, D. Ewen. *Remembering*. New York: Nervous and Mental Disease Monographs, 1947.

Cameron, D. Ewen. *General Psychotherapy: Dynamics and Procedures*, New York: Grune & Stratton, 1950.

Cameron, D. Ewen. "Frontiers of Social Psychiatry." *Psychiatric Quarterly* 20:638–655, 1946.

Cameron, D. Ewen. *Life Is for Living*, New York: The MacMillan Company, 1948.

Cameron, D. Ewen. "Dangerous men and women." Unpublished paper in the Archives of the American Psychiatric Association, Washington, D.C.

Trials of War Criminals Before The Nürnberg Military Tribunals Under Control Law No. 10, Vols. 1 & 2, Washington, D.C.: U.S. Government Printing Office, 1948.

Cameron, D. Ewen. "The social reorganization of Germany." Unpublished paper in the Archives of the American Psychiatric Association, Washington, D.C.

Cameron, D. Ewen. "Nürnberg and its significance." Unpublished paper in the Archives of the American Psychiatric Association, Washington, D.C.

Cameron, D. Ewen. "Social sciences in the building of the coming world order." Talk given on CBC Radio, May 5, 1946. Transcript in the Archives of the American Psychiatric Association, Washington, D.C.

Mitscherlich, A., and Mielke, F. *The Death Doctors*. London: Grune & Stratton, 1968.

Interviews carried out by author, 1986.

Chapter 8

Cameron, D. Ewen. *Objective and Experimental Psychiatry*. New York: The MacMillan Company, 1941.

Page, L.E.M., and Russell, R.J. "Intensified electrical convulsion therapy." *Lancet* 254:597–598, 1948.

Russell, R.J., Page, L.E.M., and Jillett, R.L. "Intensified electro-convulsive therapy." *Lancet* 265:1177–1179, 1953.

Kennedy, C.J.C., and Anchel, D. "Regressive ECT in schizophrenics refractory to other shock therapies." *Psychiatric Quarterly* 22:317–320, 1948.

Glueck, B.J., Reiss, H., and Bernard, L.E. "Regressive electric shock." *Psychiatric Quarterly* 31:117–136, 1957.

Azima, H. "Prolonged sleep treatment in mental disorders: some new psychopharmacological considerations." *Journal of Mental Science* 101:593–603, 1955.

Brickner, Richard M., Porter, Robert T., Homer, Warren S., and Hicks, Julia J. "Direct reorientation of behavior patterns in deep narcosis (narcoplexis)." *Archives of Neurology and Psychiatry* 64:165–195, 1950.

Cameron, D. Ewen. "Psychic driving." *American Journal of Psychiatry* 112:502–509, 1956.

Cameron, D. Ewen. "Psychic driving: dynamic implant." *Psychiatric Quarterly* 31:703–712, 1957.

Cameron, D. Ewen, Levy, L., and Rubenstein, Leonard. "Effects of repetition of verbal signals upon the behavior of chronic psychoneurotic patients." *Journal of Mental Science* 106:742–754, 1960.

Cameron, D. Ewen, and Pande, S.K. "Treatment of the chronic paranoid schizophrenic patient." *Canadian Medical Association Journal* 78:92–96, 1958.

Cameron, D. Ewen. "Production of differential amnesia as a factor in the treatment of schizophrenia." *Comprehensive Psychiatry* 1:26–34, 1960.

Cameron, D. Ewen, Lohrenz, J.G., and Handcock, K.A. "The depatterning treatment of schizophrenia." *Comprehensive Psychiatry* 3:65–76, 1962.

Cameron, D. Ewen, Levy, L., Rubenstein, L., and Malmo, R.B. "Repetition of verbal signals: behavioral and physiological changes." *American Journal of Psychiatry* 115:985–991, 1959.

Cameron, D. Ewen, Levy, L., Ban, T., and Rubenstein, L. "A further report on the effects of repetition of verbal signals upon human behaviour." *Canadian Psychiatric Association Journal* 6:210–221, 1961.

Hebb, D.O. *Textbook of Psychology*. Philadelphia: W.B. Saunders Co., 1972.

Solomon, P., Mendelson, Jack H., and Kubzansky, Philip E. (eds.). *Sensory Deprivation: A Symposium Held at Harvard Medical School*. Cambridge, Mass.: Harvard University Press, 1961.

Biderman, Albert D., and Zimmer, Herbert (eds.). *The Manipulation of Human Behavior*. New York: John Wiley & Sons, 1961.

Biderman, Albert D. "Communist attempts to elicit false confessions from Air Force prisoners of war." *Bulletin of the New York Academy of Medicine* 33:616–625, 1957.

Biderman, A.D. "Communist techniques of coercive interrogation." Lackland Air Force Base, Texas. Air Force Personnel and Training Research Center, December, 1956. (Development Report AFPTRC-TH-56-132, ASTIA Document #098908).

Cameron, D. Ewen, Levy, L., Ban, T., and Rubenstein, L. "Sensory deprivation: effects upon the functioning human in space systems." In *Psychological Aspects of Space Flight*. Bernard E. Flaherty (ed.), New York: Columbia University Press, 1961.

Files of the Center for National Security Studies, Washington, D.C.

Archives of the American Psychiatric Association, Washington, D.C.

Levy, L., Cameron, D.E., Aitken, R., and Cairns, B. "Observations on two psychotomimetic drugs of piperidine derivation CL 395 (Sernyl) and C1400." *American Journal of Psychiatry* 116:843–844, 1960.

Marks, *The Search for the Manchurian Candidate*.

Cameron, D.E., Levy, L., Ban, T., and Rubenstein, L. "Automation of psychotherapy." *Comprehensive Psychiatry* 5:1–14, 1964.

Interviews carried out by author, 1986.

Interviews carried out by Jay Peterzell, Center for National Security Studies in preparation for John Marks's book, 1978.

Cleghorn, R.A. "The emergence of psychiatry at McGill." *Canadian Journal of Psychiatry* 29:551–556, 1982.

Hebb, D.O. Interview with Ronald Blumer and Marian Meyer, filmmakers, July 1985.

Cameron, *Remembering*.

Blain, Daniel. Forward to *Psychotherapy in Action*.

Diagnostic and Statistical Manual of Mental Disorders (Third Edition). Washington, D.C.: American Psychiatric Association, 1980.

Chapter 9

Scheflin, Alan W., and Optin, Edward M., Jr. *The Mind Manipulators*. New York: Paddington Press, 1978.

Hunter, Edward, *Brainwashing in Red China*. New York: Vanguard Press, 1951.

Depositions of Richard Helms, Sidney Gottlieb, and John Gittinger.

Bauer, Raymond A., and Schein, Edgar H. (eds.). "Brainwashing." *Journal of Social Issues*, Vol. 13, 1957.

Biderman, Albert D. *March to Calumny: the Story of American POWs in the Korean War*. New York: The MacMillan Company, 1963.

Hinkle, Laurence E., and Wolff, Harold G. "Communist interrogation and indoctrination of 'enemies of the state.' analysis of methods used by the communist state police (a special report)." *Archives of Neurology and Psychiatry* 76:115–174, 1956.

Project MKULTRA, The CIA's Program of Research in Behavioral Modification, Joint Hearing Before the Select Committee on Intelligence and the Subcommittee on Health and Scientific Research of the Committee on Human Resources, United States Senate, Ninety-Fifth Congress, First Session, August 3, 1977. Washington, D.C.: U.S. Government Printing Office, 1977.

Miller, Merle. *Plain Speaking: An Oral Biography of Harry S. Truman*. Quoted in Scheflin and Opton, *The Mind Manipulators*, p. 233.

Project Bluebird/Artichoke from CIA Memorandum to the Select Committee, entitled "Behavioral Drugs and Testing,"

February 11, 1975. Quoted in Scheflin and Opton, *The Mind Manipulators*, p. 67.

Documents in Human Ecology File at Center for National Security Studies, Washington, D.C. Partially quoted and referenced in Marks, *The Search for the Manchurian Candidate*, p. 149.

Internal CIA Index Card Summary of each of the MK-ULTRA projects, dated October 10–14, 1956.

Opinion of George Cooper, Q.C., regarding Canadian government funding of the Allan Memorial Institute in the 1950s and 1960s. Communications and Public Affairs, Department of Justice, Ottawa, Ontario, 1986.

Interview of D.O. Hebb by Jay Peterzell on June 8, 1978.

Sargent, William. *Battle for the Mind: A Physiology of Conversion and Brainwashing*. Westport, Conn.: Greenwood Press, 1957.

Cameron, D.E., Levy, L., and Rubenstein L. "Effects of repetition of verbal signals upon the behavior of chronic psychoneurotic patients." *Journal of Mental Science* 106:742–754, 1960.

Schwartzman, A.E., and Termansen, P.E. "Intensive electroconvulsive therapy." *Canadian Psychiatric Association Journal* 12:217–218, 1967.

Chapter 13

Letters from John Marks, Joseph L. Rauh, Jr., Harvey Weinstein, Senator Pete Wilson, and Congressman Tom Lantos.

Project MKULTRA, Joint Hearing.

Allard, William. Internal CIA memorandum, October 31, 1978.

Depositions of Admiral Stansfield Turner and John Gittinger.

Penn, Judge John, U.S. District Court for the District of Columbia, December 10, 1985.

Montreal Gazette, October 31 and November 5, 1985.

Chapter 14

Homes, John. "Life with Uncle." In *The Canadian-American Relationship*. The Bissell Lectures, 1980–81. Toronto: University of Toronto Press, 1981.

Opinion of George C. Cooper, Q.C., regarding Canadian government funding of the Allan Memorial Institute in the 1950s and 1960s. Communications and Public Affairs, Department of Justice, Ottawa, Ontario, 1986.

Solomon, Mendelson, Kubzansky, *Sensory Deprivation.*

Case Study List, May 16, 1978, Center for National Security Studies, Washington, D.C.

Biderman, and Zimmer. *The Manipulation of Human Behavior.*

Brawley, Peter, and Pos, Robert. "The informational underload (sensory deprivation) model in contemporary psychiatry." *Canadian Psychiatry Association Journal* 12:105–124, 1967.

Cameron, D.E., and Rubenstein, L. "Ultraconceptual communication." In *Psychopathology of Communication.* Paul H. Hoch and Joseph Zubin (eds.). New York: Grune & Stratton, 1958, pp. 17–21.

Lehmann, Heinz E. "The place and purpose of objective methods in psychopharmacology." In *Drugs and Behavior*, Leonard Uhr and James G. Miller (eds.). New York: John Wiley & Sons, Inc., 1960, pp. 107–127.

Cole, Jonathan O., and Gerard, Ralph W. (eds.). *Psychopharmacology: Problems in Evaluation.* National Academy of Sciences, National Research Council, Washington, D.C., 1959.

Marks, *The Search for the Manchurian Candidate.*

"Tainting Canada With Shame" (letter to the editor). *Toronto Globe and Mail*, June 1986.

Baldwin, David A., and Smallwood, Frank (eds.). *Canadian American Relations: The Politics and Economics of Interdependence.* Hanover, N.H.: The Public Affairs Center, Dartmouth College, 1967.

Desbarats, Peter. *Canada Lost, Canada Found: The Search For A New Nation.* Toronto: McClelland & Stewart, 1981.

Callwood, June. *Portrait of Canada.* Garden City, N.Y.: Doubleday, 1981.

Chapter 15

Reiser, Stanley J., Dyck, Arthur J., and Curran, William J. *Ethics in Medicine: Historical Perspectives and Con-*

temporary Concerns. Cambridge, Mass.: The MIT Press, 1977.

Jones, W.H.S. *Hippocrates*. Cambridge, Mass.: The Loeb Classical Library, Harvard University Press, 1923.

Bernard, Claude. *An Introduction to the Study of Experimental Medicine* (1865). Translated by Henry C. Green. New York: Dover Publications, 1957.

World Medicine Association Bulletin 1:109–111, 1949.

Trials of War Criminals Before the Nürnberg Military Tribunals, Vols. 1 & 2. Washington, D.C.: U.S. Government Printing Office, 1948.

Ivy, Andrew C. "Nazi war crimes of a medical nature." Quoted in Reiser, Dyck, and Curran, *Ethics in Medicine*, from *Federation Bulletin* 33:133–146, 1947.

Pappworth, M.H. *Human Guinea Pigs: Experimentation on Man*. Boston, Mass.: Beacon Press, 1967.

Kater, Michael. "The burden of the past: problems of a modern historiography of physicians and medicine in Nazi Germany." Talk given at Stanford University, Department of History, April 29, 1986.

Leake, C.D. (ed.). *Percival's Medical Ethics*. Baltimore: Williams & Wilkins Co., 1927.

"American Institute of Homeopathy, Code of Ethics." Reprinted in Leonard, Charles H. *The Codes of Medical Ethics and Advertiser*. Detroit, Mich., 1878.

"Ethics governing the service of prisoners as subjects in medical experiments: report of the committee appointed by Governor Dwight H. Green." *Journal of the American Medical Association* 136:457–458, 1948.

Beecher, Henry K. "Ethics and clinical research." *New England Journal of Medicine* 274:1354–1360, 1966.

Pius XII. "The moral limits of medical research and treatment." 44 Acta Apostolicae Sedis 779–784 (1952); Rome: Proceedings of the First International Congress of Neuropathology 713–725 (1952). Translated from the French by NCWC News Service. Quoted in Katz, Jay. *Experimentation With Human Beings*. New York: Russell Sage Foundation, 1972, p. 550.

Capron, Alexander. "The law of genetic therapy." In Hamilton, M. (ed.). *The New Genetics and the Future of Man*.

Grand Rapids, Mich.: Eerdmans Publishing Co., 1971. Quoted in Katz, *Experimentation With Human Beings*.

Archives of the American Psychiatric Association, Washington, D.C.

Jones, James H. *Bad Blood: The Tuskegee Syphilis Experiment*. New York: The Free Press, 1981.

Final Report of the Tuskegee Syphilis Study Ad Hoc Advisory Panel. Washington, D.C., U.S. Public Health Service, 1973.

Katz, Jay. "Experimentation on people." *Yale Law Report* Vol. 32, Spring 1986.

Schloendorff v. Society of New York Hospital 105 N.E. 92, 93 (1914).

Fortner v. Koch, 272 Michigan 273, 261 N.W. 762 (1935).

Annas, George J., Glantz, Leonard H., Katz, J., and Barbara F. *Informed Consent to Human Experimentation: The Subject's Dilemma*. Cambridge, Mass.: Ballenger Publishing, 1977.

Katz, Jay. *The Silent World of Doctor and Patient*. New York: The Free Press, 1984.

Ladimer, Irving. "Ethical and legal aspects of medical research on human beings." 3 *Jour. Pub. Law* 467, 495–496 (1954).

The author gratefully acknowledges the assistance of James L. Turner, Esq., and Bernard Rothman, Ph.D., in reviewing some of the legal literature that is described in this chapter.

Chapter 16

Editorial, *Montreal Gazette*, February 12, 1986.

Andreev, B.V. *Sleep Therapy for the Neuroses*. Translated from Russian by Basil Hough. New York: Consultants Bureau, 1960.

Moore, Francis D. "Biologic and medical studies in human volunteer subjects—ethics and safeguards." Symposium on the Study of Drugs in Man. Part 11. Quoted in Katz, *Experimentation With Human Beings*.

Afterword

Orlikow vs. U.S., Federal Supplement 77, D.D.C., 1988.

Shenon, Philip. "CIA Near Settlement of Lawsuit By Subjects of Mind-Control Tests." *New York Times*, October 6, 1988.

CIA Brainwash settlement "a flea." Toronto Star, October 6, 1988.

"All test subjects support settlement lawyer in CIA brainwashing suit says." *Montreal Gazette*, October 6, 1988.

Shorter, Edward. "Mission of madness." *Montreal Gazette*, October 22, 1988.

Delamothe, Tony. "Unwitting victims." *British Medical Journal* 297:879–880, 1988.

Capron, Alexander M. "Human Experimentation." In *Medical Ethics*. Robert M. Veatch (ed.). Boston: Jones & Bartlett, Publishers, 1989, pp. 125–172.

Zimbardo, Philip. Personal communication. I am indebted to Professor Zimbardo for our helpful discussions around a social psychological framework for understanding physician behavior.

Lifton, Robert J. *The Nazi Doctors: Medical Killing and the Psychology of Genocide*. New York: Basic Books, 1986.

Other References

Ackroyd, Carol, Margolis, Karen, et al. *The Technology of Political Control*. London: Pluto Press, 1980.

Lifton, Robert Jay. *Thought Reform and the Psychology of Totalism: A Study of "Brainwashing" in China*. New York: W.W. Norton & Co., 1963.

McGuffin, John. *The Guinea Pigs*. Harmondsworth, UK: Penguin, 1974.

Schein, Edgar H. *Coercive Persuasion*. New York: W.W. Norton & Co., 1961.

Shallice, Tim. "The Ulster depth interrogation techniques and their relation to sensory deprivation research." *Cognition* 1:355–403, 1973.

Stover, Eric, and Nightingale, Elena O. *The Breaking of Bodies and Minds: Torture, Psychiatric Abuse, and the Health Professions*. New York, W.H. Freeman and Company, 1985.

Watson, Peter. *War on the Mind: The Military Uses and Abuses of Psychology*. New York: Basic Books, 1978.

Index